OSCEs in Psychiatry

Commissioning Editor: Michael Parkinson
Project Development Manager: Janice Urquhart
Project Manager: Frances Affleck
Designer: Erik Bigland

OSCEs in Psychiatry

Edited by

Albert Michael MRCPsych MD
Consultant Psychiatrist, Bury St. Edmunds, UK

Foreword

E. S. Paykel MD FRCP FRCPsych FMedSci
Emeritus Professor of Psychiatry, Cambridge, UK

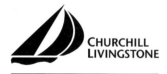

CHURCHILL
LIVINGSTONE

Edinburgh London New York Oxford Philadelphia St Louis Sydney Toronto 2004

CHURCHILL LIVINGSTONE
An imprint of Elsevier Science Limited

First published 2004

ISBN 0 443 07297 3

British Library Cataloguing in Publication Data
A catalogue record for this book is available from the British Library

Library of Congress Cataloging in Publication Data
A catalog record for this book is available from the Library of Congress

Notice
Medical knowledge is constantly changing. Standard safety precautions must be followed, but as new research and clinical experience broaden our knowledge, changes in treatment and drug therapy may become necessary or appropriate. Readers are advised to check the most current product information provided by the manufacturer of each drug to be administered to verify the recommended dose, the method and duration of administration, and contraindications. It is the responsibility of the practitioner, relying on experience and knowledge of the patient, to determine dosages and the best treatment for each individual patient. Neither the Publisher nor the author assumes any liability for any injury and/or damage to persons or property arising from this publication.
The Publisher

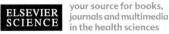
ELSEVIER
SCIENCE
your source for books,
journals and multimedia
in the health sciences
www.elsevierhealth.com

Transferred to Digital Print 2009
Printed and bound in Great Britain by
CPI Antony Rowe, Chippenham and Eastbourne

Foreword

The evolution of assessment in medical education has been a gradual one of progressive increase in reliability and validity. Medicine and its specialities are as much practical arts as systems of theory and knowledge. High standards of patient care are the ultimate goal of medical education, and assessment of clinical competence has long been regarded as a key issue for examination. The first clinical long case examination was in Cambridge in 1842. History does not record the first psychiatric clinical examination, but for many years psychiatric long cases and more recently, in some centres including Cambridge, short cases, have been an important element in examinations for medical students and for psychiatric postgraduates. Traditional examination methods are still often unreliable. Objective structured clinical examinations (OSCEs), employing real or simulated patients, are a development in response to this. They are now being introduced into the Part 1 Examination for Membership of the Royal College of Psychiatrists (MRCPsych). They lend themselves well to the short case format, usually with 10–16 stations, each with a specific task in assessment, interpretation, communication or management and with standardised assessment of the candidate. OSCEs can achieve improved reliability by standardising both variability in patients and in candidate assessment. They can be standardised in the levels of difficulty which are appropriate to a particular examination. In the right circumstances they can be close to real-life clinical situations and in addition, if using simulated patients, they can employ scenarios which would be distressing to real patients. They must be prepared with care, employing detailed oversight to ensure good scenarios, with effort devoted to training of the subjects, and attention to standardisation.

This book is intended particularly for MRCPsych Part 1 candidates. It can serve to familiarise candidates, from many different countries and previous medical school examination experiences, to the range of tasks and questions which may be encountered in the examination situation. Its content can do more than this and be valuable in its own right for skills acquisition and revision. It will also be very useful for senior medical students, for teachers both of psychiatric postgraduates and of medical students, and for general practitioners and psychiatrists seeking to brush up their skills.

Dr Michael, who has compiled and edited this book, is a very experienced psychiatric trainer, MRCPsych Course Organiser and MRCPsych Part 1 Examiner. He has previously published two valuable and successful volumes of Patient Management Problems in Psychiatry. The authors he has enlisted are experts in their fields, but close enough to the examinations, on one or both sides of the table, to tackle the devising of OSCEs and questions realistically. The OSCEs have been prepared with care.

I commend this excellent volume to prospective candidates preparing for the MRCPsych and similar examinations, to postgraduates and to students, to their teachers and to practitioners.

E S PAYKEL
Emeritus Professor of Psychiatry
University of Cambridge
24 April 2003

Preface

Objective Structured Clinical Examinations (OSCEs) are new phenomena in psychiatry. The Royal College of Psychiatrists have replaced the 'long case' or the 'Individual Patient Assessment' in Part I of their Membership Examination with OSCEs. It is likely that other colleges of psychiatrists will follow suit.

With the advent of OSCEs in psychiatry, it became evident that there were no books or other learning and teaching materials in this area. Hence, with the support of my colleagues I set out to fill this gap. We initially aimed only to give the trainees and trainers a flavour of what could be expected in OSCEs and how to prepare for them. However, by compiling a set of tasks that trainee psychiatrists routinely perform, we ended up with a book that could help not just pass the exams, but also improve clinical skills and performance.

I would like to thank the contributors who volunteered to venture into this rather unknown territory and without whose commitment and enthusiasm this book would not have materialised. I should also thank the many trainee psychiatrists who helped fine-tune the chapters.

A. M.   2003

Contributors

Jennifer Anderson BSc(Hons) MBBS MRCPsych
Specialist Registrar in Psychiatry, Cambridge, UK

Thomas H. Bak Dr med.
Research Associate, MRC – Cognition and Brain Sciences Unit, Cambridge, UK

Alison Battersby MA MB BChir MRCPsych
Specialist Registrar in Psychiatry, Cambridge, UK

John Bellhouse MB ChB MRCP MRCPsych MPhil(Cantab)
Specialist Registrar in Psychiatry, Cambridge, UK

Donald Bermingham MB BCh, BAO, MRCPsych
Consultant Psychiatrist and Clinical Tutor, Huntingdon, UK

Sadgun Bhandari, MB BS DPM MD DipNBE MRCPsych
Consultant Psychiatrist, Newham, London, UK

Catherine Corby MB BCh BAO MSc MRCPsych
Consultant Psychiatrist, Limerick, Eire

Chess Denman MB BS MRCPsych
Consultant Psychiatrist in Psychotherapy, Cambridge, UK

T. G. Dinan, MRCPsych, MD, PhD
Professor, Department of Pharmacology and Therapeutics, University College, Cork, Eire

Anthony Fernandez MBBS MD DPM MRCPsych
Assistant Director, Substance Abuse Treatment Program, McGuire Veterans Administration Medical Center, Richmond, Virginia, USA

Julian A. C. Gojer MB BS DPM MRCPsych FRCPC
Staff Psychiatrist, Law and Mental Health Program, Center for Addiction and Mental Health, Toronto; Assistant Professor of Psychiatry, University of Toronto, Canada

Neil Hunt MA MD MRCPsych
Consultant Psychiatrist, Cambridge, UK

Fiona Hynes MRCPsych MMedSci
Specialist Registrar in Psychiatry, Cambridge, UK

Furhan Iqbal MA MB BS MRCPsych
Specialist Registrar in Psychotherapy, Cambridge, UK

Rebecca Jacob MB BS DPM, MRCPsych
Specialist Registrar in Psychiatry, Cambridge, UK

Alison Jenaway BSc MB BS MRCPsych
Consultant Psychiatrist, Huntingdon, UK

Lee Kissane MA (Cantab) MB BChir MRCPsych
Specialist Registrar in Psychiatry, Cambridge, UK

Brian A. Lawlor MD FRCPI FRCPsych
Conolly Norman Professor of Old Age Psychiatry, St. James's Hospital and Trinity College, Dublin, Eire

Fernando Lazaro-Perlado LMS, MRCPsych
Specialist Registrar in Psychiatry, Cambridge; Honorary Research Fellow, Brain Injury
Rehabilitation Unit, Edgware Community Hospital, London, UK

Mervyn London MB ChB MRCPsych
Consultant Psychiatrist, Cambridge, UK

David MacDougall BSc(Hons) MB ChB MRCP(UK)
Specialist Registrar in Cardiology, Cambridge, UK

P. John Mathai MB BS DTCD DPM MD
Professor of Psychiatry and Consultant Psychiatrist, Kottayam, India

Albert Michael MRCPsych MD
Consultant Psychiatrist, Bury St. Edmunds, UK

Alex Mitchell MB BS BMedSci MRCPsych
Consultant Psychiatrist, Leicester, UK

Maria Moran MRCPsych
Honorary Lecturer in Psychiatry of the Elderly, St Patrick's and St James Hospital,
Dublin, Eire

Jacqueline E. Muller MB ChB MMed(Psychiatry)
Consultant Psychiatrist, MRC Research Unit on Anxiety and Stress Disorders,
University of Stellenbosch, Cape Town, South Africa

M. Farouk Okhai MRCPsych
Consultant Psychiatrist in Psychotherapy, Milton Keynes, UK

Christopher O'Loughlin BM BS BMedSci MRCP MRCPsych
Specialist Registrar in Psychiatry, Cambridge, UK

Nadir Omara MB BS, ABPsych, MRCPsych
Specialist Registrar in Psychiatry, Cambridge, UK

R. Raguram MB BS MD DPM MRCPsych
Professor of Psychiatry, National Institute of Mental Health and Neurosciences,
Bangalore, India

Ranga Rao MB BS DPM DMH DipNBE MD MRCPsych
Consultant Psychiatrist, University Hospital Lewisham, London; Senior Lecturer
and Course Organiser, GKT MRCPsych Course, GKT Medical School, University of
London, London, UK

Michael Robertson MB BS FRANZCP
Director, Mayo-Wesley Centre for Mental Health, Taree, New South Wales, Australia

Judy S. Rubinsztein MB ChB MRCPsych PhD
Clinical Lecturer in Psychiatry, Cambridge, UK

Barry Smith BA(Ed), CertEd Resuscitation Council (UK) Instructor
Clinical Skills and Resuscitation Training Manager, West Suffolk Hospital,
Bury St Edmunds, UK

Dan J. Stein MD, PhD
Professor of Psychiatry; Director, MRC Unit on Anxiety Disorders, University of
Stellenbosch, Cape Town, South Africa and University of Florida, Gainesville, USA

Martin Stevens FRCP FRCPsych
Consultant Psychiatrist, Ipswich, UK

Andrew Tarbuck BMBCh MA MRCPsych
Consultant in Psychiatry of Old Age, Norwich, UK

Subha N Thiyagesh MRCPsych
Clinical Lecturer, SCANLab, Academic Clinical Psychiatry, University of Sheffield, Sheffield, UK

Anthony J Vivian FRCS FRCOphth
Consultant Ophthalmologist, Cambridge and Bury St. Edmunds, UK

Marc Woodbury-Smith MBChB MPhil MRCPsych,
Clinical Research Associate, Section of Developmental Psychiatry, University of Cambridge and Ho. Specialist Registrar in Learning Disability, Cambridge, UK

Contents

Introduction

A. Michael

The long case has been the main part of clinical examinations ever since it was introduced in Cambridge in 1842. However, there have always been concerns about the effects of patient variability and examiner variability on the outcome. A study of 10, 000 medical students by the National Board of Medical Examinations, USA, found that the correlation of independent evaluations by two examiners was 25% (Hubbard et al, 1963). Leichner et al (1984) showed that the luck of the draw in selection of examiners and patients played a significant role in the outcome of postgraduate examinations in psychiatry.

OSCE stands for Objective Structured Clinical Examination. Burrows and Abrahamson (1964) first introduced OSCE in neurology clinical examinations. OSCE is a timed examination in which the candidates rotate through a circuit of examination stations. A station will usually consist of a clinical scenario with a simulated patient whom the candidate is required to interview, or a clinical problem that the candidate has to interpret or manage. The candidate's performance is observed by an examiner and assessed using a structured mark sheet.

OSCE aims to test clinical and communication skills. The examiners observe the candidate putting these skills into practice. OSCE helps examine more varied problems than the traditional long case. A greater number of examiners will reduce the effects of examiner variability. Standardised patients can improve reliability and validity. OSCE enables testing scenarios that may be distressing to the patient, e.g. bereavement and terminal illness. The stations can be adjusted to the doctor's expected skill. OSCE can have most of the engaging qualities of reality while being explicitly controlled and safe. In some centres the simulated patients give direct feedback to students. The simulated patients are more readily available than real patients.

OSCE is not just about passing examinations. It also improves clinical training and practice. It brings a sense of objectivity to the way we run our profession and helps trainees gain some insight into how the patients feel and behave. OSCE is widely used in teaching communication skills and clinical skills.

Validity of simulated patients: Expert review of stations for accuracy can ensure their content and face validity. The fact that simulated patients are rarely distinguished from real patients by the examiners or examinees in OSCE is an indirect indicator of validity. Hodges et al's (1997) finding that 80% of candidates found the stations real or very real indicates the content validity of OSCE.

Reliability or consistency of performance: Badger et al (1995) studied 13 simulated patients during 228 doctor–patient encounters over a period of 1 year. They found high intra- and inter-performance reliability even when assessments were 3 months apart. With good training, the simulated patients could be accurate and consistent in the essential features of their simulations (Vu et al, 1987). Simulated patients are able to enact their roles up to 12 times a day (Vu and Barrows, 1994).

Disadvantages of OSCE: There is a risk of OSCE assessing more textbook scenarios. OSCE may not allow the assessment of complex skills. OSCE is more expensive than traditional examinations to set up. In addition, there are training issues in setting up scenarios.

THE MRCPSych OSCE

The Royal College of Psychiatrists have replaced the long case in the Part I clinical examination with OSCE. There will be 12 *stations*. Each station has one specific task. The tasks will be appropriate for SHOs who have had a year of training in adult or old-age psychiatry. The stations test the candidate's competence in a range of clinical skills such as history taking, mental state examination, physical examination, risk assessment, data interpretation, communication, breaking bad news, counselling and patient management.

The instructions will be posted outside the station. The candidate will have 1 minute to read it. A typical station lasts 7 minutes. A bell will signal the beginning and end and there may be a warning bell 1 minute before the end. There will be a number of parallel circuits of stations at each examination centre. The stations will be the same across all the circuits and all the exam centres.

The standardised or simulated *patients* are trained actors. They follow an instruction sheet. Before the examination they are familiarised with the relevant clinical and social details. Their brief includes information on their role and the appropriate affect. They will have all the information to answer your questions appropriately. However, they will provide information only if asked. They will be instructed to stop the interaction when they hear the 'end of station bell'.

The *examiners* have standardised mark sheets. Each examiner covers all candidates attending one particular station. The mark sheet has a checklist with a score for each component of the skill assessed. The skills assessed include generic ones, such as appropriate introduction, and specific ones, such as specifying 12-hour post-lithium blood tests. Examiners do not intervene during the interview, except when they are instructed to do so, e.g., to ask for differential diagnosis.

HOW TO PASS THE OSCE

The beginning

'A bad beginning makes a bad ending' (Euripides). Hence, read the instructions carefully and understand what is required of you. Prepare a mental checklist and plan your strategy. Enter the test station ready to start, appearing confident and knowledgeable. Make a good first impression. Focus on your specified task.

Establish a rapport with the patient

Greet the patient by name, shake the patient's hand and smile. Introduce yourself warmly. Be courteous. Make the patient comfortable and at ease. Explain the purpose of the contact. Ask permission to take a history or to do an examination. Thank the patient for co-operating.

Plain language

Use appropriate, plain and understandable language and avoid medical jargon. Do not lecture to the patient or give more information than what the patient can handle. Check that the patient understands what you say. Move smoothly from one topic to another. Use illustrations and examples to promote understanding. Provide the patient with a closure.

Body language

Make use of non-verbal communication. Demonstrate an attitude of confidence, reliability and warmth. Sit at the same level as the patient. Make sure that there are no barriers such as a computer monitor between you and the patient.

Listen

Listen to the patient carefully. Show interest in the patient's story. Do not appear bored. Demonstrate that you are listening: maintain good eye contact, lean forward, keep arms uncrossed and nod appropriately. Observe the patient's body language and listen to the patient's non-verbal cues.

Questions

Start with open-ended questions. Use more open-ended rather than closed questions. Use closed questions to clarify what the patient has said and to gather factual information.

Do not repeat the same question. Do not fire a list of questions. Make the interview a conversation. Maintain the natural flow of conversation. Take clues from what the patient says.

Silence and pauses

Do not rush the patient. Use pauses and allow the patient time to think and respond. Let the patient answer one question before asking the next one.

Empathy

Remember that the patient is as human as you are. If you believe that the patient is as important as you are, you are mistaken. The patient is more important than you are. Your career depends on how well you can get on with patients and make them feel good about you. For their medical care, you are just one of the many choices. Hence, be sensitive and show warmth, empathy, concern and consideration for the patient's feelings. Try to see how you would have felt if you were in the patient's shoes. Convey your understanding and acceptance of the patient's situation. Respect the patient's dignity. Do not ignore questions from the patient. Ask permission to speak to partner/children/parents if indicated.

Interrupting the patient

Patients, and especially simulated ones, often will not give a straightforward history. The temptation to interrupt and get your work done can be irresistible.

You may use your communication skills to improve the situation; for example:

May I summarise what you have told me, so that you can check if I have got it right?

I am very much interested in what you told me just now about your mother taking an overdose. Could you tell me a bit more about it, please?

Alliance

It is best to treat the patient as an ally in tackling the problem. Hence, seek the patient's point of view and involve the patient in the management plan. Do not argue, interrupt or embarrass the patient. Avoid being judgemental or confrontational. Do not reassure prematurely or give false hope. Offer partnership and ongoing support whenever appropriate. Praise when appropriate, e.g., when the patient has managed to reduce alcohol intake or to increase physical activity.

Discuss and educate

Patients appreciate you explaining your findings, diagnosis, management plan, alternatives and prognosis and involving them in the management plan. Always enquire about the patient's understanding of the problem. Educate the patient about the importance of compliance and regarding preventive measures, lifestyle changes and risk reduction.

Summarise

Summarise periodically what the patient has said and invite him to correct you. This would make the patient feel listened to and understood. It also provides the opportunity to clarify issues with the patient.

Summarise the management plan and check that the patient has understood it.

Physical exam

You must let the patient know when you are going to begin the physical examination, explain what you plan to do and ask the patient for permission before touching him.

Do not examine the patient through the gown. You must ask the patient for permission before removing any clothing. Keep the patient draped as much as possible and ask the patient to dress as soon as the physical examination is over. Do not begin a discussion when the patient is partly undressed.

Show consideration for the patient's discomfort and pain. Do not repeat uncomfortable manoeuvres unless absolutely necessary.

Remember to assist the patient off the examination table. Explain the findings when appropriate.

In OSCE, for physical examination you may get a simulated patient or a manikin. If you get a manikin, confirm whether you are expected to speak to the manikin or to the examiner.

Closure

Encourage the patient to add information and to ask questions. Finish by thanking the patient.

Time management

Use a sensible wristwatch. Read the instruction carefully. Prepare a mental checklist of what you are going to do. Try to finish the task well in advance of the end bell. This will help accommodate any last-minute brainwaves.

When the warning bell goes and/or when you have only a minute left at the station, try to complete any remaining critical tasks and start achieving a satisfactory closure.

Remember that the simulated patients will stop the interaction when they hear the 'end of station bell'.

Preparation

Prepare or perish. Since OSCE is more predictable it is easier to prepare for. The candidates could make a list of possible OSCE tasks, i.e. history taking, examination, management, communication etc., under each topic – alcohol, anxiety, depression etc. – and make checklists and protocols for each one of them. They could undertake specific tasks in front of patients, relatives, carers, the multidisciplinary team members, trainee colleagues and consultants as part of their day-to-day work. They could use videos of interviews with patients or simulated patients, observe colleagues interviewing patients or ask colleagues to comment on one's performance. It is also important to practise time management.

HOW TO FAIL OSCE

- Do not prepare
- Turn up late for the exam
- Dress like a vagrant
- Do not read the instructions
- Do not introduce yourself to the patient
- Be arrogant, inconsiderate and discourteous
- Lecture to the patient
- Ask many questions in one go

    How are you? How is your mood? How do you feel in yourself?

- Ask only closed questions

    Do you feel down in yourself?

- Make a statement followed by a closed question

    You feel sad. Don't you?

- Touch the patient without permission
- Give premature and false reassurance
- Interrupt the patient
- Ignore clues
- Change abruptly from one topic to another
- Do not accept your ignorance
- Believe that your examiner's job is to fail you

HOW TO TRAIN THE TRAINEES

There are many ways in which educational supervisors can equip their trainees for OSCE:

- Demonstrating doing specific clinical tasks
- Observing the trainees do specific clinical tasks
- Asking the trainees to do specific tasks during the ward round. The advantage is that the trainees get over the stage fright and performance anxiety because they do the tasks in front of a bigger audience than they would come across in the examination
- Encouraging video-recorded assessments
- Making physical examination including cranial nerve examination and fundoscopy mandatory at least for all new patients.

THIS BOOK

This book describes some common OSCE stations in psychiatry. Each station includes a construct, an instruction to the candidate, and a checklist, shown in a tinted box, followed by a suggested approach. The checklist indicates the essential items and the points the scoring may be based on. Ideally, candidates should try to draw up a checklist from the information provided in the 'construct' and the 'instructions to candidate'. They could then compare it with the checklist provided. The 'suggested approach' is often a sample conversation and is very biased to the doctor's issues. Real conversations need to be reactive to the particular needs, knowledge and concerns.

We have often included more material than can usually be covered in 7 minutes. This is to cover various possible eventualities. For example, candidates are unlikely to be asked to examine all the cranial nerves in 7 minutes; however, they may be asked to examine any combination of cranial nerves.

In many chapters, the dialogues are written in full. Never try to repeat them verbatim, but take clues from them, observe other people's style and find out what works best for you. Moreover, it will be counter-productive to ask all the questions listed. With respect to dialogues, the following abbreviations are used:

C : candidate or clinician
M : medical registrar
N : neurophysiology consultant
O : on-call consultant
P : patient
R : relative or carer
S : consultant surgeon
W : William, a medical student

This book is aimed at postgraduate trainees in psychiatry as well as medical students, and postgraduates and practitioners in other clinical specialities. This would also serve as a useful aide-mémoire in the day-to-day work of clinicians dealing with mental health issues.

REFERENCES

Badger LW, DeGruy F, Hartman J et al 1995 Stability of standardised patients' performance in a study of clinical decision making. Fam Med 27: 126–133

Burrows HS, Abrahamson S 1964 The programmed patient: a technique for appraising student performance in clinical neurology. J Med Educ 39: 802–805

Hodges B, Regehr G, Hanson M et al 1997 An objective structured clinical examination for psychiatric clinical clerks. Acad Med 72: 715–721

Hubbard JP, Levitt EJ, Schumacher CF et al 1963 An objective evaluation of clinical competence. N Engl J Med 272: 1321–1328

Leichner P, Sisler GC, Harper D 1984 A study of the reliability of clinical oral examination in psychiatry. Can J Psychiat 29: 394–397

Vu NV, Steward DE, Marcy M 1987 An assessment of the consistency and accuracy of standardized patients' simulations. J Med Educ 62: 1000–1002

Vu NV, Barrows HS 1994 Use of standardized patients in clinical assessments: recent developments and measurement findings. Educ Res 23: 23–30.

FURTHER READING

Silverman J, Kurtz S, Draper D 1998 Skills for Communicating with Patients. Radcliff Press, Oxford

WEBSITES

www.cambridgecourse.com
www.rcpsych.ac.uk

1   Collateral history in frontotemporal dementia

B. Lawlor

CONSTRUCT

The candidate demonstrates knowledge of the symptoms of frontotemporal dementia (FTD), and the ability to obtain a detailed collateral history from the relative of an individual with suspected FTD.

INSTRUCTIONS TO CANDIDATE

You are asked to obtain a collateral history from the wife of a man suspected of having frontotemporal dementia.

CHECKLIST

- Empathy
- Symptoms of FTD
- Onset and progression of symptoms
- Differential diagnosis
- Relevant history: medical history, trauma, family history, premorbid personality, etc.
- Further investigations.

SUGGESTED APPROACH

C : *I am sorry to hear that your husband has not been well for a while. As part of our assessment I would like to ask you some questions about the problems he has been experiencing. Details of the type of changes you have noticed and how they have developed are very useful in situations like this.*

R : I have told our GP all I know but I will be happy to answer any questions you have.

C : *Thank you. According to the referral letter I have received, your husband has not been himself for some time. Can you describe for me how he has been?*

R : He is just not the man I married. He seems distant, doesn't take anything seriously and has no interest in things. He wouldn't bother to change his clothes unless I told him to.

C : *Tell me more about how he has changed.*

R : He can be quite moody and irritable, and has embarrassed me in public on a few occasions.

C : *I understand that this is difficult and upsetting for you. Would you mind telling me what he did?*

R : He kisses the doctor when I bring him to see her, and he talks to strangers on the bus, asking them personal questions.

C : *When did this all begin?*

Was the onset sudden or gradual?

Since you first noticed changes in your husband, have things got worse or stayed the same, or do his symptoms fluctuate?

R : Looking back, it all began about 3 years ago. He became irritable and over-talkative. Recently, he was caught shoplifting. Since then he has been getting worse.

Enquire about further symptoms of frontotemporal dementia.

Behavioural disorder
- Self-neglect, lack of grooming
- Disinhibition, sexualised behaviour, aggression
- Distractibility, impulsivity, impersistence
- Lack of insight
- Do a brief risk assessment.

Affective symptoms
- Depression, anxiety
- Emotional unconcern, indifference
- Lack of spontaneity
- Hypochondriasis, bizarre somatic preoccupation.

Speech disorder
- Progressive reduction of speech
- Stereotypy of speech i.e. repetition of limited repertoire of words, phrases or themes
- Echolalia and perseveration
- Late mutism.

Physical symptoms and signs
- Early incontinence
- Rigidity, tremor, akinesia.

Consider the differential diagnosis
- Frontal lobe syndrome secondary to vascular lesion, head trauma or other space-occupying lesion: enquire about onset and risk factors
- Other dementias, e.g. Alzheimer's disease: enquire about cognitive symptoms
- Substance misuse
- Mood disorders: enquire about pervasive mood change and associated symptoms
- Psychotic disorder.

R : What do you think it might be doctor?

C : *At this point, we are gathering information to help us make a diagnosis. This interview is only one part of the assessment. I would like to see your husband next and then order some tests. I will discuss the outcome of the assessment with you both then. We are considering a number of possibilities. Problems with the front part of the brain would explain some of your husband's symptoms, or his symptoms may be explained by a depressive illness.*

2 Elicit an alcohol history

M. London

CONSTRUCT

The candidate demonstrates the ability to elicit a detailed alcohol history.

INSTRUCTIONS TO CANDIDATE

A 40-year-old labourer was admitted to the medical ward with chest pain. Routine blood tests showed increased GGT and MCV. The physicians have requested an assessment. Elicit an alcohol history.

CHECKLIST

- Introduce the topic tactfully
- Typical day/week
- History
- Edwards and Gross (1976) criteria: tolerance, withdrawal, relief drinking, stereotyped pattern, compulsion, primacy, rapid reinstatement
- CAGE: cut down, annoyed, guilt, eye opener
- Risk factors
- Complications
- Treatment
- Insight
- Summary
- Motivation.

SUGGESTED APPROACH

An alcohol assessment should serve as the first step in management. Avoid the temptation to be critical or judgemental.

Introduction

C : *I gather that you are in the hospital because of chest pain. I have been asked to see you to discuss your blood test results. Is that all right with you?*

Some of your tests show that your liver is under strain. What do you think might be affecting your liver?

Have you had any problems with your liver in the past?

Sometimes alcohol can affect the liver. Can you tell me about your drinking habits?

Typical day/week

C : *How often do you drink?*

Let us go through a typical day – when would you have the first drink?

How much would you drink on a typical day?

What about weekends?

What do you usually drink?
What else would you drink?
Do you usually drink alone or in company?
How many units of alcohol would you have in a week?

Help the patient calculate the units per week.

History
Ask about when the patient first tasted alcohol, started drinking occasionally and regularly at weekends, evenings, lunchtimes and in the mornings.

Tolerance
C : *What is the maximum you have drunk in a day?*
How much can you drink without feeling drunk?
Nowadays, do you need more alcohol to get drunk than what you needed last year?

Withdrawal
Ask about shakes, retching, sweating and waking up with these.
C : *How often do you cut yourself shaving?*
What happens if you miss your drink?
What would happen if you go without a drink for a day or two?
Were there times when you were seeing or hearing things when you could not have your usual amount of alcohol?
When was the first time you noticed this?

Relief drinking
C : *Do you need a drink the first thing in the morning to steady your nerves?* (**eye opener**)
Do you have to gulp the first few drinks of the day?

Stereotyped pattern
C : *Do you always drink in the same pub?*
Do you always drink with the same company?
Do you usually drink regularly or in sprees?

Compulsion
C : *Do you sometimes crave a drink?*
Do you find it hard to stop drinking once you start?

Other CAGE questions
C : *Do you feel that you have to cut down on your drinking?*
Do people annoy you by criticising your drinking?
Do you feel guilty about your drinking?

Risk factors for alcohol abuse
Occupation, premorbid personality, psychiatric history, family history of alcoholism.

C : *What types of work have you done over the year?*

Complications

Ask about family, social life, work and financial problems and problems with the law, e.g. drunk driving, drunk and disorderly behaviour, fights while drunk.

C : *Have you done anything when you were drunk but later regretted?*

Health problems

Ask about health problems, accidents and injuries to self and others, depression, anxiety, suicidal ideation/behaviour, memory blackouts etc.

C : *Did you ever wake up in the morning unable to remember what happened the night before when you had been drinking as usual?*

Do you use any drugs?

Primacy

C : *How did these [the above] problems affect your drinking?*

How often do you miss family and social commitments for drinking?

Treatment and rapid reinstatement

Ask about treatment and periods of abstinence.

C : *What helped you keep off drinks?*

What made you start drinking again?

When you restarted, how long did it take before you were back to your usual level?

Insight

C : *Well, do you feel you have a problem with alcohol?*

Enquire about the good and bad things about his drinking, about what he thinks will happen if he continues to drink, and what he wants to do about his drinking.

Summary

C : *Let me summarise what we discussed. You drink approximately x units of alcohol a week. This is y times the safe limit. Alcohol makes you feel relaxed and gives you company. On the other side you can't miss your drink even for a day. You tend to get severe shakes and sweating. Alcohol seems to be affecting your physical health, especially your liver. Alcohol is causing problems in your relationship, work, finances and friendships. Alcohol also tends to get you into trouble. You have been concerned about your drinking and you want to do something about it. Am I correct?*

Motivation

C : *What would you like to do?*

Have you ever thought of giving it up completely?

What do you think will happen if you give up completely?

I will give you some reading material. I would like you to think about it and discuss it with your family and friends. I will make an appointment to see you and your partner together to discuss plans. Is that all right with you?

Elicit symptoms of mania

3

T. G. Dinan

CONSTRUCT

The candidate demonstrates the ability to establish a rapport with a patient and elicit the symptoms of mania, while keeping in control of the interview.

INSTRUCTIONS TO CANDIDATE

You have been asked to see a 40-year-old man in the Accident and Emergency Department. The A&E sister is concerned about his irritability and agitation. Assess him for symptoms of mania.

CHECKLIST

- Remain in control of the interview, while being calm and courteous
- Focus on the task
- Mood – elation, irritability
- Biological features – energy, sleep, appetite, libido
- Interests
- Grandiose ideas, delusions
- Other psychotic symptoms
- Speed of thought
- Impulsivity
- Social activity
- Judgement and insight
- Summary.

SUGGESTED APPROACH

To start with, it may be useful to allow the patient to talk uninterrupted for a short while. Premature interruption may increase the eagerness to speak. Hence, wait for natural breaks. Look for any themes arising. Grab opportunities to guide the patient by reflecting, summarising or paraphrasing the patient's words.

If he deviates from the topic, bring him back tactfully. If he has pressure of speech and/or flight of ideas, interrupt politely and firmly and move on to closed questions. Use closed questions more often than usual, especially if he is over-talkative.

Avoid confrontation. Do not become frustrated, angry and impatient. If the patient is annoyed and/or agitated, acknowledge this and reassure him.

C : *You are obviously upset. Tell me how I can help you.*

I appreciate what you are saying. We have only a few minutes and I must ask you a few questions. I will listen to you once we have finished my questions.

Mood

Elation

C : *How do you feel in yourself?*
How are you in your spirits?
Can you describe what it's like, please?
Do you feel very cheerful or high?
Do you feel on top of the world?
What about feeling low?

Irritability

C : *How do you get on with people?*
Do they annoy you?
Do you lose your temper easily?
Do you feel irritable or angry?
Could you describe what happens when people irritate you?

Biological features

Energy

C : *What is your energy level like?*
Have you felt tired in recent days?
Has everything speeded up?
Have you been working harder than usual lately?

Sleep

C : *How has your sleep been lately?*
Do you feel that you need much less sleep?

Appetite

C : *How has your appetite been lately?*
Have you lost weight recently?
Have you noticed your clothes becoming too big for you?

Libido

C : *How has your interest in sex been lately?*

Interests

C : *Could you tell me about your interests?*
Have you developed any new interests lately?
Have you taken on any new commitments?

Grandiosity

C : *How do you see yourself compared to others?*
Do you feel more self-confident than usual?
Do you have any special abilities or powers that others do not have?
Is there a special purpose or mission in your life?
Do you have any special plans?
Are you specially chosen?
How do you see the future?

Other psychotic symptoms

Enquire about delusions of persecution and reference, religious experiences, auditory hallucinations of God or important people talking, visual hallucinations etc.

Speed of thought

C : *Has there been any change in your thinking lately?*
Have you noticed that your thoughts speed up?
Do you find your thoughts racing in your mind?
Do you have more ideas than usual?
Do you have more ideas than you can handle?
Do things seem to go too slowly for you?

Impulsivity

C : *Have you been buying a lot of things?*
Have you been in trouble with the police lately?
Have you been drinking more alcohol than usual?
Have you been experimenting with any illicit drugs lately?

Social activity

C : *Have you made any new friends lately?*
Have you been making more telephone calls than usual?
Have you been writing to people?

Judgement and insight

C : *Is your family concerned about you?*
Do you regret anything you did lately?
Was there any reason why things went a bit wrong for you recently?
Would you agree that you are not usually like this?
What would you think if I said that you are like this because you are ill?
I think you will get back to your normal self if you have some rest and some medication. Would you agree?
What would you like me to do for you?

Summary

C : *I think you have been feeling unusually well in yourself. You have been more irritable than usual. You have been unable to sleep or look after yourself properly. Your thoughts have speeded up. You have been experiencing and doing things that you would not usually do. You have been spending more money and drinking more alcohol than usual. You have been getting into trouble. I know that it will be difficult for you to see our point, but we all feel that you are not well and that you need some rest and some medication.*

Assess suitability for Interpersonal Psychotherapy

4

M. Robertson

CONSTRUCT

The candidate demonstrates the ability to assess the suitability of a patient with depression for Interpersonal Psychotherapy (IPT).

INSTRUCTIONS TO CANDIDATE

A consultant psychiatrist colleague referred a 40-year-old man to your service for IPT. He has been depressed for about a year. He showed little response to antidepressant drugs. Please assess his suitability for the treatment.

CHECKLIST

- Establish the interpersonal contributing factors to the depression
- Establish extent of prior knowledge of IPT
- Enquire about previous psychotherapies
- Identify potential interpersonal problem areas
- Explain IPT problem areas
- Explain the rationale for IPT
- Discuss contractual issues.

SUGGESTED APPROACH

C : *I understand your consultant has referred you for Interpersonal Psychotherapy because the medication has not been helpful so far.*

P : That's right.

C : *Perhaps we could start by you telling me a little of the background of how you came to be depressed. I am particularly interested in any relationship difficulties that occurred around that time.*

P : Well, I seemed to take my father's death very badly. He died about 18 months ago without any warning. I just haven't been able to get over it.

C : *I am sorry. Were you and your father close?*

P : Yes. He was my main support person. I always went to him for advice.

C : *I see. Is your mother still alive?*

P : Yes.

C : *How have things been between you and her since your father died?*

P : Well, she has become more dependent on my wife and me. She is even talking about wanting to move in with us.

C : *How does your wife feel about this?*

P : Well, she and I have not been getting on very well since our daughter left for university.

C : *Could you tell me more about that?*

P : Well, she left for university 3 months ago and she is now 300 miles away.

C : *Were you and your daughter close?*

P : Yes we were, although she was closer to her mother than me.

C : *How have things changed at home since your daughter left for university?*

P : Well, that, and combined with the problems with my mother, certainly made for tense times.

C : *So, to summarise, it appears that your depression started when your father died. It has certainly continued in the context of other problems, including difficulties with your mother, problems at home with your wife and also adjusting to life after your daughter left for university.*

P : Yes, I suppose that is right.

C : *Could I ask what you know about Interpersonal Psychotherapy?*

P : The only thing I know is that it is a talking treatment that looks at relationships.

C : *Well, it appears that your medication has not been helpful in fully relieving your depression. It is certainly clear from scientific evidence that talking treatments help to improve responses to medication and vice versa.*

P : I see.

C : *Have you had any other forms of talking treatments or counselling?*

P : Yes, I spoke to the practice nurse for a couple of sessions. She tried to get me to keep a diary of my activities and encouraged me to do more pleasant things.

C : *Did you find that helped things?*

P : Not really.

C : *Were there any difficulties in that treatment?*

P : I found her to be a little bit pushy and I did not really see the point of what she was trying to do.

C : *Did you have an opportunity to ask her about it?*

P : Not really, no.

C : *Perhaps I could ask, do you think that your current relationship difficulties might be important to how you are feeling?*

P : Well, yes, since we have been talking about it.

C : *Well, it seems that you became depressed at the time that your father died suddenly, which is certainly understandable. It does seem that things have worsened because of other problems, such as the problems in your marriage, the problems adjusting after your daughter left for university and the ongoing problems with your mother.*

P : Well, now that you have pointed it out, yes I do see that.

C : *Do you think there could be other factors that might be important, such as work, stress, money problems, your health – that kind of thing?*

P : No, not really. I have usually been quite well and we have been well off.

C : *So it does seem that relationships are the major problem?*

P : Yes it is.

C : *Perhaps I could explain what Interpersonal Psychotherapy actually involves.*

Firstly, it is a focused treatment and is time limited. We will probably meet for between 12 and 16 sessions and each session will have a very specific focus. In your case, we will try to identify the important relationship difficulties that are relevant to your depression.

P : Okay.

C : *In Interpersonal Psychotherapy, we try to categorise these as one of four problems. The first problem area is Interpersonal Disputes, such as arguments, disagreements or disappointments. Do you think there have been any of those in your life?*

P : Well, I suspect the problems with my wife could be seen as disputes.

C : *Well, that would make sense. The second problem area we talk about in IPT is Role Transitions. In Role Transitions there have been changes of circumstances that may be very obvious, such as retirement or changing jobs, or they may be very subtle, such as adjusting to life after a child leaves home or a change in the nature of a relationship. Role transitions are often tricky to identify, as people are often not aware of the change. Do you see any role transitions in your life?*

P : Well, I guess my daughter leaving home would fit that.

C : *Yes, I suppose it would, but we would need to look at that more closely. The third problem we talk about is that of Grief. In IPT, when we talk of grief as a problem area, we acknowledge that a person has not got over the death of a loved one. Some other people use grief to mean other things, but it appears that your father's sudden death seemed to trigger the depression. This would be quite relevant to you.*

P : Well, absolutely.

C : *The final area in IPT is Interpersonal Deficits or Interpersonal Sensitivity. This relates to people's inability to establish and maintain supportive relationships. It is very common for people who feel depressed to underestimate their ability to do this. Often people who are not depressed also experience this deficit. This might become more apparent as the treatment progresses.*

Well, that was the IPT in a nutshell. Do you think that it may help with your depression?

P : Yes, the way you explain it does help.

C : *I will give you some reading material that describes in more detail what we have discussed.*

5 Mini Mental State Examination

M. Moran

CONSTRUCT

The candidate demonstrates the ability to put the patient at ease and perform the MMSE in a sensitive and non-threatening manner. The candidate also demonstrates awareness of deafness or visual impairment that may affect performance.

INSTRUCTIONS TO CANDIDATE

Perform the MMSE on Mrs Smith, who is 78 years old.

CHECKLIST

- Rapport and empathy
- Explain the assessment and check the patient's ability to hear, see and understand you
- Inquire about relevant facts, eg, educational level and occupational history
- Administer and score the MMSE
- Appropriate response to an incorrect answer

SUGGESTED APPROACH

C : *My name is _____ . Your doctor has asked me to see you for a check-up. I will start with some questions about your background, if that is alright.*

P : What? [It appears that she cannot hear.]

Candidate moves slightly closer, and speaks a little louder.

C : *Can you hear me now?*

P : Yes.

C : *Let me know if you cannot hear me. I have some questions for you about your background. How old are you? How long have you been retired? What did you work at?*

P : I am 78 years of age. I was a teacher, and have been retired for nearly 15 years. I went to school until I was 17, and then went on to teacher training college.

C : *Do you have any problems with your memory?*

P : No, not that I am aware of.

C : *Do you mind if I ask you some questions to test your memory?*

P : No, not at all.

Temporal orientation

C : *What year is it?*
Season?
Month?
Date?
Day?

Score one point for each correct answer. If it is near transition between seasons you may accept either season, and be aware of geographical differences in terminology.

Spatial orientation

C : *Where are we now?*
What country?
County?
City/town?
Building?
Floor of building?

Score one point for each correct answer.

Registration

C : *Listen carefully. I am going to say three words. I want you to say them out loud after me. Ready? Here they are: APPLE, PENNY, TABLE.*

Allow 1 second between each word. Score 1 point for each correct word. The order does not matter. This score is based on this first trial only. However, if the individual does not successfully repeat all three words on the first trial, repeat them up to a maximum of five times until the patient is able to say all three words back to you. Then say 'Now keep those words in mind. I am going to ask you to say them again in a few minutes.'

Attention and concentration

Serial 7's

C : *I would like you to subtract 7 from 100. Then keep subtracting 7 from each answer until I tell you to stop. What is 100 take away 7? … Keep going.*

Score 1 point for each correct answer, up to a maximum of five subtractions. The answer is correct if it is exactly 7 less than the previous answer, regardless of whether the previous answer was correct.

WORLD backwards

C : *Could you spell WORLD?*

Correct any misspelling.

C : *Now could you spell it backwards?*

One point is given for each letter in the correct order, e.g. dlrow = 5, dlorw = 3.

Recall

Recall should be tested 5 minutes after presenting the words.

C : *What were the three words I asked you to remember?*

Do not prompt. If the individual has difficulty, be encouraging but do not give hints. Be empathic if the patient cannot recall them, and focus on her positive answers.

Score 1 point for each correct word, order does not matter.

Naming

Show the patient a pen and then a watch and ask her to name them.

Score 1 point for each object (or part of object) correctly identified.

Repetition

C : *I want you to repeat exactly what I say. 'No ifs, ands or buts.'*

Articulate it so that all the plural endings are clear and audible. You may repeat the phrase if the individual has difficulty hearing or understanding you, up to a maximum of five times, but the score should be based only on the first attempt to repeat the phrase.

Score 1 point if the patient repeats the entire phrase correctly, on the first attempt.

Comprehension

C : *Listen carefully, because I am going to ask you to do something. Take this paper in your right hand, fold it in half and put it on the floor.* [Use the left hand if the right is impaired.]

Score 1 point if she takes the paper in the right hand, 1 point if she folds it roughly in half, and 1 point if she places it on the floor.

Reading

C : *Please read this and do what it says.*

Show her 'CLOSE YOUR EYES' in large print. She gets one point only if she closes her eyes. If she cannot read she gets zero points, but provide an explanation.

Writing

Give the patient a blank piece of paper and a pen. Ask her to write a sentence. If she does not respond, ask her to write about the weather.

Give the maximum score of 1 point only if she writes a comprehensible sentence that contains a subject and a verb. Ignore errors in grammar or spelling.

Drawing

C : *Please copy this design.*

Place a picture of the interlocking pentagons in front of the patient. She scores 1 point if she draws two five-sided figures that intersect to form a four-sided figure. The two figures do not have to be perfect pentagons but they must have five sides.

C : *Thank you for your co-operation.*

If the patient did well:

C : *You did well on that test. While you didn't get everything right, your result was within the normal range.*

If the patient did badly:

C : *How do you feel you did?*

P : Not well doctor, I couldn't remember the things you wanted me to.

C : *Yes, Mrs Smith, you did have some difficulties in certain areas, but you did fine on other questions. There are several possible reasons why you had these difficulties, and I would like to do some more tests to find out the reasons in your case. When I have these test results we can have another meeting to discuss treatment for these problems.*

Do you have any questions for me?

P : No thanks, doctor. I will wait until we get the tests.

6 Assess capacity to consent

J. Bellhouse

CONSTRUCT

The candidate demonstrates the ability to assess capacity to consent and to liaise with the surgical team.

INSTRUCTIONS TO CANDIDATE

Mr King is a 69-year-old man under the care of a general surgical team in your hospital. He was admitted 2 days ago with malaise and vomiting, for investigation. Examination and investigations suggest bowel obstruction. He is refusing to sign the consent form for exploratory surgery. The surgical team has asked for him to be 'sectioned' to enable the operation to go ahead. Assess his capacity to consent or withhold consent to the operation and communicate your findings to the consultant surgeon.

CHECKLIST

- Speak to the surgeons to ascertain the facts of the case
- Introduce yourself to the patient and explain your role
- Assess his capacity to consent/withhold consent for the operation
- If he lacks capacity, ascertain the mental disorder responsible for this
- Inform the surgical team of your opinion and explain their options.

SUGGESTED APPROACH

Speak to the surgeons to ascertain the facts of the case

Find out the reason for admission, the current problem, the surgical procedure needed, the risks of surgery, the prognosis with surgery and without surgery.

Introduce yourself to the patient and explain your role

C : *Hello, Mr King, I am Dr ____, one of the psychiatric doctors in this hospital. Mr S, the consultant surgeon looking after you at the moment, has asked me to see you to help decide what we should do about a problem that has arisen with your treatment. I understand that Mr S believes you need an operation to find out why your bowel is blocked and to fix the problem and that you do not wish to have the operation. Is this so?*

The patient's understanding of the overall problem

C : *Tell me what you understand about the problems you are having at the moment.*
What have you been told is wrong with your tummy?
Have the surgeons told you why you feel so ill and cannot hold down any food?
Have you ever had an operation before?

The patient's understanding of the nature of the proposed procedure

C : *Do you know what the surgeons think needs to happen?*

What have they told you about the anaesthetic that would be used?

Have they told you that the operation might leave your tummy looking different to what it does now?

Have they told you that you may need a bag for going to the toilet after the operation?

The patient's understanding of the purpose of the procedure

C : *Why do you think you need an operation?*

Why do the surgeons think you need an operation?

The patient's understanding of the risks of the procedure

C : *Have the surgeons told you about the risks of having the operation?*

Do you think that it will be painful?

Is it possible that you may die?

Do you think that it may leave you with scars?

The patient's understanding of the risks of not having the procedure

C : *What do you think will happen if nothing is done?*

Do you think that you will get better if nothing is done?

Having ascertained the patient's level of understanding, give the relevant information where the patient does not understand it and ask again. Give the information in simple, clear terms and on a bit-by-bit basis, then assess whether he has understood it.

Does the patient believe the above information?

C : *Do you believe there is a blockage in your bowel?*

Why don't you believe this?

What do you think is the problem?

Is the patient able to weigh the information in order to come to a decision?

C : *Can you tell me the pros and cons of the operation?*

Tell me why you have decided not to have the operation.

Ascertain the final decision

C : *We have had a detailed discussion about why the surgical team feel you need the operation. Tell me, what do you think you are going to say now to having the operation?*

Why is that?

Are you sure?

If the patient lacks the capacity to make the decision, take a focused psychiatric history and perform Mental State Examination.

Thank the patient and explain that you need to speak to the surgeon in order to decide the best thing to do now.

Throughout the interview, the patient has been unable to focus on what you are saying, appears unfocused and episodically in pain. Mental State Examination reveals problems with orientation in place, poor attention and memory deficits. His case notes reveal a low level of plasma sodium (126 mmol/l). The clinical picture is one of delirium due to his medical condition which significantly impinges on his capacity.

Explain this to Mr S.

C : *I have seen Mr King. In my opinion he lacks the capacity to withhold consent to his operation as he cannot understand the relevant information, retain it or weigh it in the balance to come to a decision.*

S : Will you write in the notes that you are happy for me to go ahead?

C : *I will record my opinion in his case notes but, as the operating surgeon, the final decision as to whether to proceed will be yours, taking into account the best interests of the patient.*

S : Shouldn't he be put on a section?

C : *The Mental Health Act (1983) would only allow us to admit him to a psychiatric hospital for assessment or treatment. It would give us no authority to proceed with surgery, which occurs on the same legal basis irrespective of whether he is detained under the Mental Health Act or not. Currently his physical condition must take priority. However, I will review his mental state postoperatively.*

S : His only relative is a daughter in Australia, and it might be a week before she comes to sign the consent form. What are we going to do in the meantime?

C : *As the patient is an adult, no one else has the power to consent on his behalf. The daughter should be consulted as a matter of good practice, by telephone if necessary. However, the final decision to treat an adult lacking the capacity to consent remains with the treating doctor, and takes into account the best interests of the patient.*

NOTES AND REFERENCES

Definition of Capacity

Re C (Adult: Refusal of Medical Treatment) 1994 All England Law Reports 819

Law Commission 1995 Mental Incapacity: A Summary of the Law Commission's Recommendations (LC231). Stationery Office, London

Best interests

Re F (Mental Patient: Sterilisation) 1990 4 Butterworth's Medical Law Review 1.

Overviews

Bellhouse J et al 2001 Decision making capacity in adults: its assessment in clinical practice. Adv Psychiat Treat 7: 294–301

Kennedy I, Grubb A 2000 Medical Law. Butterworths, Oxford

Elicit delusions

R. Raguram

CONSTRUCT

The candidate demonstrates the ability to establish a rapport with a patient presenting with psychotic symptoms and to elicit delusions.

INSTRUCTIONS TO CANDIDATE

A GP has referred a patient for assessment of psychotic symptoms. Elicit delusions, if any.

CHECKLIST

- Introduce the topic tactfully
- Start with open questions and then move on to closed questions
- Persecution
- Reference
- Grandiosity
- Guilt
- Nihilism
- Jealousy
- Delusional mood
- Control and passivity experiences
- Thought alienation and thought block
- Other delusions
- Conviction, elaboration, effects and coping
- Try to differentiate delusions from overvalued ideas
- Conclusion.

SUGGESTED APPROACH

Introduction

C : *Your doctor asked me to see you because he has been concerned about you. I would like to ask you some questions. Some of them may appear a bit strange. These are questions which we ask everybody who comes to the hospital. Is that all right with you?*

I gather that you have been through a lot of stress and strain recently. When under stress some people find their imagination playing tricks on them. Have you had any such experiences?

Do you have any ideas that your family and friends do not agree with?

Do you have any worries or concerns?

I am afraid I did not make myself clear enough. Let me put it in a different way.

Persecution

C : *How do you get on with others?*
   Do they annoy you?
   Are you afraid of them?
   Would you trust most people you know?
   Are there some people who try to harm you or make your life miserable?
   Do you think that someone is watching, following or spying on you?
   Is there a plot to harm you?

Reference

C : *Do people talk behind your back?*
   What do they say?
   Do people drop hints about you or say things with a special meaning?
   Do things seem specially arranged for you?
   Does everyone gossip about you?
   Do you see any reference to yourself on the TV or in the newspapers?

Grandiosity

C : *How do you see yourself compared to others?*
   How confident do you feel in yourself?
   Do you have any special powers or abilities?
   Is there a special purpose or mission in your life?
   What about special plans?
   Do you feel people are organising things specially to help you?
   Are you specially chosen in any way?

Guilt

C : *Do you have any regrets?*
   Do you feel you have done something wrong?
   Do you feel you deserve punishment?
   Do you feel guilty?
   Do you feel that you might cause harm to others?

Nihilism

Enquire about being doomed, being a pauper, intestines being blocked etc.

C : *Do you feel something terrible has happened or will happen to you?*
   How do you see the future?

Hypochondriasis

This might involve cancer, HIV/AIDS etc.

C : *How's your health?*
   Are you concerned that you might have a serious illness?

Jealousy

C : *Can you tell me about your relationship?*

Do you feel that your partner reciprocates your loyalty?

[If he admits not to] *Have you been trying to produce some evidence?*

Delusional mood

C : *Do you have a feeling that something strange is going on, which concerned you, but you did not know what it is?*

Control and Passivity experiences

C : *Is there anyone trying to control you?*

Do you feel under the control of some force other than yourself? (As though you are a robot or a zombie without a will of your own?)

Do they force you to think, say or do things?

Do they change the way you feel in yourself?

Can you resist them?

Thought alienation

C : *Are you able to think clearly?*

Is there any interference with your thoughts?

Usually whatever one thinks is his own thoughts. Has it been the case with you too?

Do others put or force their thoughts into your mind? [Thought insertion]

Can people read your mind?

Does everyone know what's in your mind, as if your thoughts are broadcast?

Could someone take your thoughts out of your head? [Thought withdrawal]

Would that leave your mind empty or blank?

Others

C : *Do you feel that an impostor has replaced a familiar person?*

Are you a very religious person?

Are you in a special relationship?

Do you have any other concerns that we have not discussed?

Conviction, explanation, effects, coping

Do not be satisfied with a 'Yes' answer. Probe, elaborate and clarify. Ask who does these things, why and how.

C : *How do you know that this is the explanation?*

Could it be your imagination?

What do your family and friends think about this problem?

Ask how it affects him – does it make him annoyed, irritable, frightened etc.? Ask how he copes, what he has done and what he intends to do about these things.

Conclusion

Summarise, invite corrections, acknowledge the distress and thank the patient.

8 Elicit symptoms of obsessive-compulsive disorder

J. E. Muller D. J. Stein

CONSTRUCT

The candidate demonstrates the ability to elicit symptoms and signs of obsessive-compulsive disorder (OCD) and screen for the presence of OCD-spectrum disorders.

INSTRUCTIONS TO CANDIDATE

A GP has referred a 24-year-old man to you who has severely chapped hands due to repeated hand washing. Elicit features of OCD and screen for OCD-spectrum disorders.

CHECKLIST

- Obsessions
- Compulsions
- Insight
- Symptom severity
- Onset and course of symptoms
- OCD symptom dimensions
- OCD spectrum disorders
- Co-morbidity
- Feedback.

SUGGESTED APPROACH

C : *Your doctor asked me to see you because he was worried about the condition of your hands. Could you tell me more about this?*

P : I guess they look like this because of all the washing. You see, somehow I keep thinking that my hands are dirty, so I wash them over and over again.

C : *How do you mean 'dirty'?*

P : I keep thinking there are germs on my hands and under my nails and that I might spread them or get ill if I'm not careful.

C : *So these must be pretty contagious and dangerous germs?*

P : I know, it sounds crazy! I know that we all carry germs all the time, so my worries don't make sense. But I can't keep them away.

C : *How do you make certain that there aren't any more germs under your nails?*

P : I use an antibacterial soap, but I lose track of how many times I wash. It must be more than 30 times a day, because I think about the germs almost all of the time.

Obsessions

C : *Let me ask you more about these thoughts [images or impulses in other cases].*

Do they keep coming back to you even when you try not to have them?

Do you find them intrusive?

How do they make you to feel in yourself?

Compulsions

C : *What about ignoring or getting rid of these thoughts?*

Do you try to neutralise these thoughts in any way?

Do you wash your hands [mental rituals in other cases] repeatedly because you keep thinking they are dirty?

What about showering or bathing, or cleaning household/other objects excessively?

Does washing make you feel less anxious?

How do you decide when to stop washing?

Do you check anything to make sure there is no dirt or germs?

Are there things you do to prevent coming into contact with dirt or germs?

Insight

C : *Do you think these obsessions/compulsions are excessive or unreasonable?*

What would happen if you didn't wash?

How certain are you about this?

Do these thoughts come from your own mind?

Symptom severity (including distress, avoidance, control) and impairment

Enquire about time taken and the distress caused by the symptoms and their impact on and interference with work, studies, relationships or home life.

C : *How hard do you try to resist the obsessions/compulsions?*

How much control do you have over the obsessions/compulsions?

Are there situations related to obsessions/compulsions that you avoid?

Are there things that you don't do because of the obsessions/compulsions?

Onset and course of symptoms

Enquire about onset, precipitating factors (e.g. streptococcal infection), course and when they started affecting day-to-day life.

OCD symptom dimensions

Contamination (already covered)

Aggressive

C : *Do you fear that you might harm yourself or others in any way?*

What do you do to prevent this happening?

Sexual/religious

C : *Do you have forbidden or seemingly perverse sexual thoughts/images/impulses?*

Are you overly concerned with what is morally right and wrong or blasphemy?

Do you repeatedly check anything because of this?

What about needing to tell or confess?

Symmetry/ordering/counting/arranging

C : *Are there things you have to do in a very precise or exact way?*

Do you count or order things to get them in just the right way or symmetrically?

Hoarding/collecting

C : *Do you save/collect things that are of little sentimental or monetary value?*

Do you have trouble throwing things away?

Somatic

C : *Are there aspects of your body or health that you are concerned about?*

Do you mirror-check or ask for reassurance repeatedly?

Miscellaneous

C : *Are you a superstitious person?*

Do you have lucky/unlucky numbers or colours that have a special significance?

OCD spectrum disorders

See somatic OCD symptom dimension for body dysmorphic disorder and hypochondriasis. Enquire about Tourette's disorder, trichotillomania, stereotypic movement disorder, (skin picking, nail biting, scratching, body rocking etc.)

C : *Have you had sudden movements or made sounds that you were unable to control? What about things like eye blinking, grunting, sniffing or snorting?*

How often do these movements or sounds occur?

Have you ever pulled out your hair, leaving bald patches or leaving you with thin hair?

Do you have repetitive, seemingly driven behaviours such as nail biting?

Co-morbidity

Enquire about misuse of painkillers, tranquillisers, alcohol, drugs and any beneficial effects. Rule out depression, other anxiety disorders, eating disorders, head injury, seizure disorder etc.

Feedback

C : *Is there anything else that you think is important for us to talk about? Do you have any questions?*

P : No, not at the moment.

C : *What you describe fits in with an illness called obsessive-compulsive disorder, or OCD. Although people are often very ashamed of their symptoms, feeling that no one else could suffer from these kinds of uncontrollable thoughts/actions, it is actually very common and affects 2–3% of the population during their lifetime. People used to think of OCD as the result of unconscious conflict, but we increasingly think of OCD as a neuropsychiatric condition that involves particular brain circuits. Fortunately, treatments are often effective – we use both medication and psychotherapy. I will give you some reading material on OCD and its treatment. How does that sound?*

P : Relieved to know that I'm not the only person with this, and that there's some hope for treatment.

Management of lithium toxicity

9

A. Mitchell

CONSTRUCT

The candidate demonstrates an understanding of the adverse effects of lithium carbonate and the ability to discuss the management of lithium overdose with a colleague.

INSTRUCTIONS TO CANDIDATE

A 40-year-old woman with known bipolar affective disorder presents to A&E complaining of difficulty walking, slurred speech and severe shakes. She reports that she had taken three times the prescribed dose of lithium tablets 4 hours ago. The on-call medical registrar assessed the patient, ordered a lithium level and then contacted you.

CHECKLIST

- Communication
- Therapeutic and toxic lithium levels
- Toxic effects of lithium
- Side effects of lithium
- Lithium monitoring.

SUGGESTED APPROACH

M: *I have just seen a 40-year-old woman who has taken too many lithium tablets. Can you take her over in psychiatry?*

C : I think I need a bit more information before I can proceed. You say she took too many lithium tablets. Could you specify the type and amount of lithium she has taken? I would also like to know more about her clinical presentation, especially if she has features of toxicity. Moreover, I am not clear as to why she took too many tablets.

M: *She says she was confused and took too many tablets accidentally. She brought in the bottles with her. It appears that she took 2400 mg of lithium carbonate 4 hours ago. Her lithium level now is 2.8 mEq/l and she is complaining only of slurred speech and shakes. What do you make of that?*

C : A lithium level of 2.8 is dangerously high. The normal therapeutic range is 0.6–1.2. However, the sample was taken at 4 hours post ingestion rather than 12 hours. Thus, we have a high peak level. Therefore, we should recheck the level with a trough sample to obtain a standardised value. Toxicity usually occurs at levels greater than 2.0 mEq/l and the clinical picture is suggestive of toxicity. I suggest admitting the patient for medical observation.

M: *I am not sure if these symptoms are related to lithium overdose. What other features should I look out for?*

33

C : The toxic effects of lithium mainly involve the CNS, although systemic symptoms also occur. There is often lethargy progressing to reduced consciousness in severe cases. Speech is affected with dysarthria. There will be ataxia and coarsening of peripheral tremor. There may be hyperreflexia and occasionally fasciculations, chorea or myoclonus. Systemically the patient may have diarrhoea or seizures. QT prolongation can occur. If untreated, renal failure is a recognised complication. In this case, if the slurred speech, course tremor and the ataxic gait started after the lithium ingestion there is every reason to suspect lithium toxicity.

M : *Are there any vulnerability factors that make lithium toxicity more likely?*

C : Lithium is excreted by the kidneys in exchange for sodium. Therefore, anything that interferes with renal function e.g. kidney disease, low-sodium diet, drug interactions, reduced volume distribution due to dehydration and electrolyte imbalance, would increase the risk of developing toxicity. Older age and organic brain disease are also considered risk factors.

M : *I am not sure what treatment is required, even if we did admit her.*

C : If any of the risk factors we discussed are present, we need to treat them.

In mild cases, observation and monitoring of vital functions and blood chemistry may be sufficient and no other treatment may be necessary.

However, after a recent overdose, gastric lavage rather than activated charcoal is helpful. Haemodialysis or peritoneal dialysis is the treatment of choice for severe intoxication. Complications are usually completely reversible, but a minority experience residual cerebellar dysfunction or cognitive dysfunction. QT prolongation can also be a factor in those with cardiovascular disease or on other relevant medication like antihistamines. Thus there is good reason to consider a medical admission.

M : *Out of interest, what are the long-term non-toxic effects of lithium?*

C : The most frequent adverse effects are weight gain, fine tremor and increased thirst. About a fifth of patients experience skin problems such as alopecia or acne, nausea/vomiting, goitre or renal changes. Less common again, but still important, are peripheral oedema and benign ECG changes.

M : *When should I restart lithium and discharge her?*

C : Once the 12-hour lithium level has dropped below 1.2 mEq/l it will be safe to restart lithium, provided there is no renal damage and provided the patient is happy to continue with lithium.

You should double check that the patient has not taken this intentionally. If she has taken an intentional overdose, I want to review her before discharge.

You mentioned that the patient was confused about her correct dosage. Please explore this. If she is having problems with her medication regimen, we need to adjust this.

M : *How can we minimise similar problems in the future?*

C : Regarding future management, I would continue the arrangements for serum lithium estimations once every 3–6 months once a stable lithium level is achieved.

For all patients, before commencing lithium treatment, I would explain the common side effects and toxic effects so that they would be more likely to report them if they did occur. I would remind them that the tendency to weight gain can be offset with improved diet and exercise and particularly by avoiding high-calorie drinks. I would explain that certain side effects, for example tremors, can be managed by further medication. If a patient is unhappy with lithium or if the side effects are intolerable, I would be happy to try alternative mood stabilisers.

I would also give all patients written information on bipolar affective disorder and lithium therapy, before commencing lithium treatment.

REFERENCES

Jefferson JW, Greist JH 2000 Lithium. In Sadock BJ, Sadock V (eds) Kaplan & Sadock's Comprehensive Textbook of Psychiatry (7th edn). Lippincott Williams & Wilkins, Philadelphia

El-Mallakh RS 1986 Acute lithium neurotoxicity. *Psychiat Dev* 4: 311–328

10 | Management of agoraphobia

J. Anderson

CONSTRUCT

The candidate demonstrates the ability to establish a rapport with the patient and to explain the management of agoraphobia with panic attacks.

INSTRUCTIONS TO CANDIDATE

A 40-year-old woman is referred by her GP with a 1-year history of agoraphobia with panic attacks. Explain the management options to her.

CHECKLIST

- Explain options
- Education
- Pharmacological
- Psychological: graded exposure and cognitive therapy
- Role of partner/relative
- Advantages of combined approaches over individual ones
- Prognosis.

SUGGESTED APPROACH

C : *I gather that you have a fear of going out alone and you get panic attacks. Your doctor has diagnosed you to have agoraphobia with panic attacks and you want to discuss the treatment. Am I correct?*

P : Yes, you are.

C : *Well, it is very important that you know about your illness and the treatments available. This would help us work together, and make the treatment a partnership between us and thus get the best results. Would you agree?*

P : I think so.

C : *Good. We may not be able to go through all the issues today. I will be happy to see you again if you have more questions. Please feel free to interrupt and to ask me questions.*

P : All right.

C : *Agoraphobia and panic attacks are common problems. There are a number of different treatments available. If you have any strong views or preferences regarding your treatment, we will try to accommodate them. There are three aspects to treatment. They are education, psychological treatments and medication. Which one shall we talk about first?*

P : I think we will start with education. That sounds simple.

C : *Education may sound simple, but education for you and your family is the most important part of the treatment. You and your family need to know about the nature of the illness, what keeps it going and how to tackle it. Your family needs information about how best to help you.*

Have you heard of any medication for agoraphobia?

P : I know people who take Valium and who drink to control their nerves.

C : *People do, unfortunately. There are two main types of medication: benzodiazepines and antidepressants. Benzodiazepines, for example Valium, which you mentioned, start working very quickly and can be useful in the short term. However, soon you will need to increase the dose to have the same effect, and you may become dependent on them. Moreover, they do not help the underlying problems. Since you have had this for about a year, benzodiazepines are not the answer.*

However, antidepressants would be a very good option. We start them at a low dose and increase gradually. It may take up to 8 weeks for it to start working. Once you feel better, you will have to continue the medication for about 6 months, if not longer. Then we have to taper it off gradually and stop. They are not addictive.

P : But I am not depressed doctor!

C : *That is a very good point. Antidepressant drugs are useful in a number of different conditions. We use antidepressants to treat a variety of conditions including anxiety, obsessions, agoraphobia and panic attacks, not just depression. They work by modifying certain chemicals in the brain. These chemical problems are common to all these disorders.*

Do you know of any psychological treatments for your sort of problems?

P : Do you mean counselling?

C : *No, not exactly. The psychological treatments are of two types. They both last between 8 and 16 weeks.*

The first is graded exposure with relaxation. First, we will teach you relaxation exercises to help you control your anxiety and panic. Then we make a list of things you find difficult to face. We order them from the least difficult to the most difficult. Then you start facing the easiest situation, while managing to relax. When you feel comfortable with that situation, you then go onto the next one. You will have to do this daily. You may find it easier to face the situations, for example going out, with a member of the family or a member of the mental health team.

P : Can you explain those exercises please?

C : *Muscle relaxation helps because muscles become tense when you are afraid or anxious. You can learn how to relax different muscles in your body and focus on the ones that become particularly tense, so that you are then able to keep them relaxed when facing the feared situation.*

In addition, learning controlled breathing would also help.

P : How would that help?

C : *Well, to put if briefly, when we panic our body gets into a fight-or-flight mode. We breathe very fast in order to get more oxygen to our muscles, for example to be able to run away or fight. Consequently we breathe out carbon dioxide. This makes the carbon dioxide level in our bodies low and produces strange physical sensations like dizziness, tingling in our hands and feet and breathlessness. When people feel breathless they breathe faster. Can you see how this will make your symptoms worse?*

P : Yes, so if I breathe properly I will feel better?

C : *Yes, if you breathe normally, your symptoms won't be as severe.*

P : What is the other treatment you mentioned?

C : *There is another form of psychological treatment using cognitive techniques. It explores your thoughts when you are anticipating the event and while feeling anxious. It looks at the links between your thoughts, emotions, physical symptoms and behaviour, as these seem to maintain the problem.*

P : You mentioned my partner. What can he do?

C : *Your partner has an important role in the treatment. He will need to learn how the therapy works, so that he is able to support, motivate and help you to tackle problems that keep the illness going. He could support you and accompany you with the exposure treatments. Therefore, it will be very helpful if he can be involved.*

P : Will I get better?

C : *Most people with agoraphobia improve to a great extent, especially when education, medication and psychological treatments are used together. Those who are in a stable and supportive relationship do better. However, most people do not become completely well. They continue to experience mild anxiety in the feared situations. The outcome is not so good especially for those who have chronic life stresses. Relapses are common. If you have a relapse, it would be best if you contact us sooner rather than later.*

Do you have any more questions?

P : No, but what shall I do now?

C : *I will give you a fact sheet describing the nature of agoraphobia and panic attacks and all the treatments available, and also a self-help manual. I would like you to read it, think about it and discuss it with your partner. I will see you again in 2 weeks time. I would like to see you with your partner if that is all right with you.*

Out-patient review in schizophrenia

A. Battersby

CONSTRUCT

The candidate demonstrates the ability to do a routine out-patient review of a patient with schizophrenia.

INSTRUCTIONS TO CANDIDATE

You are asked to see a 45-year-old man with a 20-year history of paranoid schizophrenia. He occasionally has persecutory delusions and third person hallucinations. The patient is attending your clinic for a routine 6-monthly follow-up appointment.

CHECKLIST

- Communication
- Biological functions
- Current circumstances
- Alcohol and drug misuse
- Medication, side effects
- Mental State Examination
- Risk of harm to self and others
- Education
- Termination.

SUGGESTED APPROACH

Greet the patient appropriately. Introduce yourself.

C : *I would like to find out how you have been lately. Please feel free to interrupt me if needed. Is that all right with you?*

Is there anything in particular we need to discuss or anything you are concerned about?

How have you been keeping in yourself generally?

Tell me how you have been getting on with things generally.

Has there been anything worrying you?

These open-ended questions may reveal thought disorder and abnormalities of speech.

Biological functions and current circumstances

Often, these things matter more to the patient than the psychopathology. They also give an indication about negative symptoms.

- Sleep, appetite, energy
- Accommodation, benefits, occupation, occupational therapy
- Day-to-day activities, relationships, socialization, attending day centre etc.
- Contact with the key worker and other mental health workers
- Alcohol and drug abuse.

Medication

C : *Could you tell me what medication you are taking?*

Enquire about his compliance with the medication and about his views on the type and dose of the medication.

Ask about side effects such as stiffness, shakes, restlessness, weight changes and sexual side effects.

Mental State Examination

- Appearance and behaviour
  - Look for evidence of self-neglect
- Speech
- Mood
  - Rule out depressive symptoms
- Risk of harm to self
- Thought content
  - Persecutory and other delusions
- Perceptual anomalies
  - Auditory hallucinations
- Risk of harm to others
  - Has the patient had any thoughts of harming anyone?
  - If yes, clarify whom, why, how, plans, intent etc.
- Cognition
- Insight.

Physical examination

Look for extrapyramidal symptoms.

Weigh the patient if appropriate.

Education

C : *Is there anything you want to ask me?*

What do you think about your treatment?

I am sure you know that you need to take your medication regularly in order to remain well. Seeing your key worker regularly and attending the occupational therapy, the day centre and the fitness centre will keep you even better.

If the patient has a substance misuse problem, remind him of the risks.

Enquire if he already has or wishes to have some written information about his illness and its treatment.

Termination

C : *I have looked at your medical records. I think you have moved a long way from how you were 6 months ago. I am sure you have worked hard to make things better. Shall I arrange an appointment for you in 6 months' time? I will be happy to see you earlier if required. You are welcome to come with a friend or a relative.*

Is there anything else we need to talk about? Thank you very much for talking to me.

Explain the need for antipsychotic medication

12

F. Hynes

CONSTRUCT

The candidate demonstrates the ability to establish a rapport with a young man suffering from schizophrenia, explain the need for medication and discuss the patient's concerns about medication.

INSTRUCTIONS TO CANDIDATE

A 19-year-old man admitted 4 weeks ago with a diagnosis of first episode of schizophrenia has been treated with an atypical antipsychotic and is now preparing for discharge. He wants to discuss with you the need for continued medication.

CHECKLIST

- Diagnosis
- Need for medication: treatment and prophylaxis
- Other treatments
- How medication works
- Side effects
- Depot medication.

SUGGESTED APPROACH

C : *Hello, I am ____ . I understand you want to speak to me about your medication.*

P : Yes, I have been taking these tablets since I was admitted. When I go home I don't really want to keep on taking tablets.

C : *To begin with, could you tell me the reason why you have been taking the tablets? Has anyone discussed your diagnosis with you?*

P : Yes, the consultant said I had schizophrenia.

C : *What does that mean to you?*

P : Well, it is when people hear voices and do strange things.

C : *You are correct. Schizophrenia is a serious mental illness. It affects thinking, emotions and behaviour. It affects one person in every 100 people. The illness often lasts for a long time and can be very disabling. However, with the new treatments the outlook is much better. The medication helps control the symptoms of schizophrenia and helps you cope better with stresses and will protect you from relapses.*

P : The medication has done its job. The voices don't bother me so much now. So, I think I should stop the tablets and get on with things.

C : *It is good that the tablets have helped you feel better and you want to get on with your life. However, I think we need to talk about the medication.*

When you were unwell and distressed by symptoms such as hearing voices and feeling persecuted, the medication helped you feel calmer. Then over the next few weeks

41

the medication controlled and stopped these symptoms and got you better. Medication is an important first step, which makes it possible for you to make use of other sorts of help and support.

It is equally important that you remain well. Medication helps prevent relapses and lessens the severity of the relapses. Therefore, it is important to keep taking medication even when you feel well.

P : What will happen if I stop the medication?

C : *If you stop the medication, the symptoms will come back. They do not come back immediately, but usually within about 6 months. Therefore, it is especially important to continue medication after discharge when you are trying to adapt back into things, as this can be a stressful time.*

P : Does the medication not cure schizophrenia?

C : *There is no cure for schizophrenia. Medicines help control the symptoms and to stay well. In addition, we offer other things to help you to have the best chance of getting better. This would include help with accommodation, assessing what your current skills are and what jobs you can do, getting you in touch with groups who provide work training and arrange voluntary work. When people become unwell and get admitted to hospital they lose touch with their friends and give up their hobbies and interests. The day centres offer opportunities to meet other people and provide a range of activities including 'keep-fit' and creative pursuits.*

P : How does medication work?

C : *Certain chemical messengers in the brain control our thoughts, feelings and behaviour. The most important ones are called dopamine and serotonin. Schizophrenia is associated with changes in the levels or actions of these messengers. The medication helps correct these changes.*

P : Will I become addicted to these tablets?

C : *No, they are not addictive.*

P : Do they have any side effects? I have noticed some people on the ward with funny movements. I don't want to end up like them.

C : *Like any medication, they also have side effects. There are two types of drugs used in the treatment of schizophrenia.*

The older drugs can cause shakiness and stiffness. Some people feel restless and one in 20 gets lasting movements of the mouth and tongue. Some people can feel flat, sleepy and slow.

You are now taking one of the newer drugs. They are more likely to help with the so-called negative symptoms including social withdrawal and lack of motivation. However, they are more likely to cause weight gain and sexual side effects.

P : I know another patient on the ward who complains of feeling flat all the time.

C : *In some people, the feeling flat may be due to the illness itself. We call them negative symptoms. The newer drugs are more likely to help with these. Some others feel flat because they are depressed. For them, taking antidepressant drugs in addition to the antipsychotic drugs can be helpful.*

When people feel flat because of the medication, we either change the type or dose of medication or try to counter the side effects using other drugs.

P : I don't have any side effects now. What will I do if I start getting them later?

C : *One of the psychiatrists and another member of the Community Mental Health Team will be seeing you on a regular basis. If you have any worries, you can discuss them with one of them. There is a variety of different antipsychotic drugs available. So we can try readjusting the dose or changing the type of drug or add another drug to counter the side effects.*

P : It will not be easy to remember to take tablets every day at home.

C : *It may be best to make taking the medication part of your daily routine, perhaps one of the things you do before going to bed. We can get you a dosset box, which could help remind you to take your medication.*

Some people find it hard to take tablets every day and they find it easier to take the medication as an injection. They are called depot injections. They are given once every 2, 3 or 4 weeks. Currently there is only one atypical drug available as a long-acting injection.

Is there anything else you would like to ask?

P : Not really.

C : *To sum up, medication is very important in your treatment as it helps you get better, to remain well and to prevent relapses. If you have any concerns about your medication, please feel free to discuss them with one of us. You are always welcome to come with a friend or a relative. I can give you a drug information leaflet, which explains the medication and its side effects.*

P : Thank you.

13 | Call the on-call consultant

R. Jacob

CONSTRUCT
The candidate demonstrates the ability to formulate a management plan for a patient who wants to leave the hospital and to discuss the plan with the on-call consultant.

INSTRUCTIONS TO CANDIDATE
You are the on-call SHO for a Friday night. A 25-year-old man suffering from bipolar affective disorder was admitted informally during the day, with a relapse of hypomania, due to non-compliance with his mood stabiliser, lithium. He has a history of dangerous driving, assaulting his family members and assaulting nursing staff during his previous episodes. At 8.00 p.m. the nursing staff informed you that the patient has become aggressive and agitated and that he wants to leave the hospital as he feels he doesn't have a mental illness. On assessment, he has grandiose and persecutory ideas. Formulate your management plan and get approval from the on-call consultant by telephone.

CHECKLIST
- History: diagnosis, current medication and past psychiatric history
- Assess the mental state and the current need for hospital treatment
- Risk assessment: risk to the patient, staff and others
- Formulate a management plan
- Awareness of the Mental Health Act
- Emergency management plan
- Follow-up action on Section 5(2)
- Discuss with the consultant.

SUGGESTED APPROACH
C : *Hello Dr X, I am Dr ____, the on-call SHO for psychiatry. I am sorry to disturb you. I gather that you are the on-call consultant. I need to discuss a patient's case with you.*

O : Why didn't you call the daytime consultant? Can't you wait till Monday?

C : *I am sorry Dr X. The problem arose only now. It will be risky to wait.*

O : Yes, go on, be quick.

C : *There is a patient named BP. He is a 25-year-old man with a history of bipolar affective disorder. He was admitted earlier today with a hypomania. He is attempting to leave the ward.*

O : Is the patient currently on a section?

C : *No, he was admitted informally earlier today.*

O : What do we know of the patient's history?

C : *He has a long history of bipolar affective disorder. He was apparently non-compliant with his mood stabiliser and has now had a relapse of hypomania.*

O : What will happen if you let him go?

C : *The problem is that he has a history of dangerous driving, assaulting his family and assaulting the nursing staff.*

O : What is his mental state like?

C : *He is aggressive and agitated. He has grandiose and persecutory ideas. He is threatening to leave. The nurses feel quite threatened by his behaviour.*

O : Have you reviewed his medical records?

C : *Yes. He has a 5-year history of bipolar disorder. His relapses have been due to non-compliance with medication. He has a history of violent behaviour when ill.*

O : Was he admitted compulsorily before?

C : *All previous admissions were under the Mental Health Act.*

O : Why was he admitted informally this time?

C : *Apparently, he was only mildly hypomanic and he was happy for a voluntary admission.*

O : That's fine. What medication is he on?

C : *He was on lithium but presently is prescribed only antipsychotics – haloperidol. He has refused all oral medication since his admission.*

O : What do you want to do?

C : *I think it will be too risky to let him go and therefore it would be appropriate to detain him under Section 5(2) of the Mental Health Act.*

O : What else?

C : *I would suggest rapid tranquillisation with parenteral lorazepam and haloperidol. I will arrange for him to be nursed in the side room and for special observation.*

O : That sounds fine to me. What next?

C : *I will review him tomorrow before I leave and hand over to the weekend on-call SHO. On Monday, I will inform the patient's RMO so that an assessment under the Mental Health Act can be done within 72 hours.*

O : What section do you think he will consider?

C : *Section 3, for treatment, I suppose.*

O : That's correct. Any other problems?

C : *No. Thanks.*

14 Elicit symptoms of post-traumatic stress disorder

C. Corby

CONSTRUCT

The candidate demonstrates the ability to elicit the history and symptoms of post-traumatic stress disorder (PTSD) and assess their severity and complications.

INSTRUCTIONS TO CANDIDATE

The GP has referred a 40-year-old businessman to you for assessment. He presented to the GP with a history of increasing difficulty coping. Elicit the history and features of PTSD, its severity and complications.

CHECKLIST

- History of trauma
- Onset and duration of symptoms
- Persistent re-experiencing
- Avoidance
- Hyperarousal
- Impaired social functioning
- Co-morbidity
- Treatment and outcome
- Pre-morbid personality, past history
- Insight, expectations
- Feedback.

SUGGESTED APPROACH

C : *What brings you to the clinic today?*

P : Nightmares.

C : *Could you tell me more about the nightmares, please?*

P : They are very scary. I can't even think about them.

C : *I understand, but it would be useful if you could tell me exactly what happens in your nightmares.*

P : It's about my car hitting and killing a pedestrian.

C : *Does that remind you of something?*

P : Yes, I hit a man on the road a year ago. It was not my fault.

Trauma

Find out about when it happened, how scary it was, any injuries, any head injury etc. Enquire about any blame, litigation, court cases and their outcome.

C : *I know it is very distressing, but could you describe the accident, please?*

Do you have any difficulties remembering parts of the accident?

How long after the accident did the nightmares start?

Persistent re-experiencing

Recollections, flashbacks, dreams, as if reliving the event, distress on exposure, physiological reactivity.

C : *How often do you think about the accident?*

Do these thoughts seem to force their way into your mind?

Do you sometimes feel as if the accident is happening again?

Do you get flashbacks?

What would happen if you hear about an accident?

Do you get palpitations or sweating or shaking?

Avoidance

Avoiding thoughts, places and people. Amnesia, decreased interest, restricted affect, sense of an aforeshortened future.

C : *Do you deliberately try to avoid thinking about accidents?*

How would you do that?

Have you been to the place where the accident happened?

How do you travel these days?

How hard is it for you to talk about the accident?

Have there been any changes in your feelings generally?

Can you, for example, experience loving feelings?

How do you see the future?

Are there any other activities that you avoid?

Hyperarousal

Sleep disturbance, anger, impaired concentration, hypervigilance, exaggerated startle response, aggression towards self, others and property, trouble with the law etc.

C : *Do you startle easily?*

Do you feel on edge all the time?

Tell me about your sleep, please.

Are you sometimes afraid to go to sleep?

How is your concentration?

How has your memory been lately?

Tell me about your temper, please.

Distress, impaired social functioning

C : *How has all this been affecting you?*

Have others commented that you have changed in some way since the accident?

How do you spend your time these days?

How do you feel in yourself generally?

Enquire about effect on family, social life and work.

Premorbid personality, past history

C : *Before all this happened, what sort of a person were you?*

How did you cope with stress?

Did you have any mental health problems before the accident?

Is there anyone in your family who has a mental health problem?

Did this accident bring back any previous bad memories?

Co-morbidity

Enquire about depressive symptoms, guilt feelings, suicidal thoughts, anxiety symptoms unrelated to the trauma, obsessive symptoms, somatisation, physical health, caffeine, alcohol and drug use.

C : *What other problems have you been having since the accident?*

Treatment

Ask about any treatments he had and the outcome.

Insight and expectations

C : *What do you think is the problem?*

What do you think we should do?

Feedback

C : *Shall I tell you what I think is the problem? You seem to have what we call a post-traumatic stress disorder, or PTSD for short. This is an illness which often follows a severe trauma. People suffering from PTSD often have flashbacks and nightmares and they feel on edge. They often try hard to avoid thinking about the trauma. Sometimes this can be so distressing that people may become depressed or find ways to block out their symptoms. Some people abuse alcohol or drugs for this reason. Do you have any questions for me?*

P : Is there anything we can do about this?

C : *PTSD is a treatable illness. We can treat your problem with medication or psychological methods or both. Medication involves taking antidepressant drugs. Psychological treatments include anxiety management, relaxation training, cognitive behavioural therapy and eye movement desensitisation. The most important fact is that your illness is treatable.*

Could you repeat what we discussed?

P : No, I can't remember.

C : *That is all right. I will give you some written information on PTSD. Please go through it and discuss it with your family and friends. I will make an appointment for you in a week's time to discuss treatment. You are welcome to bring someone with you.*

Examine cranial nerves

15

T. Bak

CONSTRUCT

The candidate demonstrates the ability to examine the cranial nerves and explain to the patient the purpose, procedure and findings.

INSTRUCTIONS TO CANDIDATE

Examine the cranial nerves of this middle-aged person, who presents with a 3-month history of headaches. Do not do fundoscopy.

CHECKLIST

- Remember the cranial nerves and their functions
- *Check for the appropriate instruments.*

   I Olfactory
   – smell

   II Optic
   – vision, light reflex and accommodation

   III Oculomotor
   – eye movements – other than lateral rectus and superior oblique

   IV Trochlear
   – eye movements – superior oblique

   VI Abducent
   – eye movements – lateral rectus
   A pen torch, Snellen chart, near vision chart or a newspaper, disposable neurological pins

   V Trigeminal
   – motor – muscles of mastication: wasting, jaw jerk
   – sensory – each division: sharp, blunt and fine touch, corneal reflex
   Disposable neurological pins, cotton wool

   VII Facial
   – upper face
   – lower face

   VIII Vestibulocochlear
   – hearing
   – balance

   IX, X Glossopharyngeal, vagus
   – motor
   – swallowing
   – ?gag reflex
   Tongue depressor, glass of water

XI Accessory
- trapezius
- sternocleidomastoid

XII Hypoglossal
- tongue

Pen torch

SUGGESTED APPROACH

C : *I have been asked to test the nerves on your head. Is that all right with you?*

I Olfactory

Explain that you want to test his ability to smell. Check that the nasal passages are clear by asking him to blow the nostrils separately.

C : *Would you close your eyes and close your left nostril please?*

Bring the scent to the right nostril.

C : *Could you tell me if you get any smell?*

If the patient answers correctly, inform him. Then ask him to close the right nostril and bring another scent to his left nostril.

C : *Could you try again please?*

Give feedback if he answers correctly.

II Optic

Visual acuity (VA)

Check distance and near VA in each eye separately with the other eye closed. The person should wear glasses/contact lenses if usually worn.

C : *Now I would like to check your eyes. Could you close your left eye and read that card with your right eye. Start from the top, please.*

Check distance VA using a Snellen chart held 6 metres away from the patient. Each line of letters on the Snellen chart has a number, 60, 36, 24, 18, 12, 9 and 6. This indicates the distance in metres a normally sighted person could read that line. The normal distance VA is 6/6, i.e. the person can read the last line; 6/9 to 6/60 indicate increasing impairment.

Record the distance VA. Repeat the same on the other eye.

For near VA, use a near vision chart. If it is not available, grade visual acuity as follows:

A: Can read ordinary typeface
B: Can read newspaper or magazine headlines
C: Can count fingers
D: Can see hand waving
E: Can distinguish between light and dark.

Visual fields
Test visual fields by confrontation using fingers in each of the four quadrants.

Visual inattention
Test using bilateral simultaneous stimulation. You and the patient must keep looking straight ahead. Find your blind spot by using a pin. Start laterally and bring it in slowly until it disappears and then reappears.

III, IV, VI Oculomotor, Trochlear, Abducent
Inspect the eyes for any abnormality

Check pupil size, shape and symmetry.

Look for squint – divergent or convergent.

Eye movements
Fix the patient's head with one hand. Ask the patient to look up, down, to the left and the right, with both eyes open.

Ask the patient to follow your finger with his eyes and to report if double vision occurs.

Use the H pattern for individual muscles.

Diplopia
Ask about seeing double at any stage while checking eye movements.

Diplopia is maximal when looking in the direction of the weak muscle. The false image is less clear than the true image. The false image is displaced farthest in the direction of the weak muscle.

Record the direction in which double vision occurs and where maximal separation of images occurs.

Ask the patient to close one eye at a time to find out which eye produces the false image.

Nystagmus
Look for nystagmus on normal and extreme gaze. Check if it is vertical, horizontal or rotatory and its direction.

Nystagmus is named according to the direction of the fast movement. It is maximal when looking in the direction of the fast movement.

The fast movement is towards central lesions e.g. cerebellar, and away from peripheral lesions, e.g. vestibular.

Pupillary reflexes
Light reflex
If a light is directed at one eye, both pupils will constrict. The constriction of the pupil on the stimulated eye is called the direct light reflex. The constriction of the other pupil is called the consensual or indirect light reflex.

Test for direct and indirect pupillary light reflex using a pen torch.

Accommodation reflex

Ask the patient to look at a distant object and then quickly at your finger 20–30 cm from the patient's nose. Look for convergence, slight ptosis and pupillary constriction.

V Trigeminal nerve

Sensory functions

Test each division separately and compare the left and the right sides.

Pinprick

Use disposable neurological pins. Do not use venepuncture needles.

Demonstrate the sensation to the patient on the sternum.

C : *This is sharp and this is blunt. Please close your eyes and say 'blunt' or 'sharp' when I touch you with one of them.*

Fine touch

Use fine touch using cotton wool. Do not tickle or stroke.

Corneal reflex

C : *I want to touch your eye with this. Can you look up in the ceiling for me please?*

With a small wisp of cotton wool drawn to a point, touch the exposed lower cornea lightly. Approach from the side and not from the front. Normally the patient will blink. Look for direct and indirect corneal reflexes.

Motor functions

Muscles of mastication, i.e. temporalis, masseters and pterygoids.

Wasting

Examine for hollowing around the temporal arch

C : *Can you clench your teeth please?*

Look at the masseters and temporalis. Palpate to see their bulk.

Test the pterygoids.

C : *Can you open your mouth when I press on your chin, please?*

Jaw jerk

C : *Please open your mouth lightly. I will place my finger on your chin and tap on my finger. This will not hurt.*

Place your index finger over the point of the jaw. Strike your finger gently in a downward motion using the knee hammer. The muscles contract and the jaws close in a positive jaw jerk.

VII Facial nerve

The facial nerve is predominantly motor. The upper part of the face has bilateral innervation. Hence, an upper motor neurone lesion will spare the forehead. A lower motor neurone lesion will affect the whole side.

Look for any facial asymmetry and flattening of the nasolabial fold.

Upper part of face

C : *Can you furrow your forehead please?*
Now, please raise your eyebrows.
Please close your eyes tightly.

Lower part of face

C : *Please blow out your cheeks.*
Would you whistle please?
Please show me your teeth.

VIII Vestibulocochlear

Ask the patient to repeat a word whispered in each ear.

Rhomberg's test

Ask the patient to stand up with eyes open and heels together.

Marked swaying suggests cerebellar disease.

Ask the patient to close his eyes.

Swaying suggests posterior column involvement.

IX, X Glossopharyngeal, Vagus

The glossopharyngeal is predominantly sensory to the palate. It can be tested by gently touching the pharyngeal arches on either side. The gag reflex is too variable to be useful.

The vagus is predominantly motor. Palatal weakness causes a nasal quality to speech.

C : *Could you please say 'aah'.*

Observe the uvula with a torch. Use a tongue depressor if needed. Weakness on one side will pull the uvula to the other side from its normal central position.

Swallowing

Give the patient a glass of water and ask him to drink. Look for lips closing, larynx elevating and any spluttering or coughing.

XI Accessory

The accessory nerve supplies sternomastoid and trapezius.

Look for wasting.

C : *Please push your head forwards against my hand.*

The sternomastoids will contract.

C : *Now, turn your head sideways against my hand.*

The opposite sternomastoid contracts.

C : *Please shrug this shoulder and I will press it down.*

Observe elevation of trapezius. Try both sides.

C : *Now push my hand away with this cheek.*

Try both sides.

XII Hypoglossal

C : *Please open your mouth. I want to look at your tongue.*

Using a torch, look for wasting and fasciculation.

C : *Please put your tongue out.*

It will deviate to the side of weakness.

Conclusion

Explain the findings to the patient, invite questions and thank the patient.

NB: Be prepared to examine any single or combination of cranial nerves, e.g. cranial nerves II–VIII, cranial nerve VII, cranial nerves of the eye.

When examining the optic nerve, examine the fundi unless you are specifically asked not to.

Elicit history of opiate use

A. Fernandez

CONSTRUCT
The candidate demonstrates ability to establish a rapport with a patient and elicit history of opiate use, the complications and the treatments he had and his degree of insight and motivation.

INSTRUCTIONS TO CANDIDATE
A young man who abuses opiates has presented himself to the Drug Treatment Centre asking for help. Elicit history of opiate use.

CHECKLIST
- Use motivational interview style
- Types of drugs
- Opiate use: heroin and other opiates, onset, progression, route etc.
- Tolerance, withdrawal symptoms and withdrawal relief
- Complications: social, medical
- Treatment
- Insight, motivation, support systems
- Background
- Summary and conclusion
- Do not be critical, judgemental or disrespectful.

NB: Patients may be evasive and may minimise problems. They may exaggerate drug use in order to get substitute prescriptions. They may have agendas other than sorting out the drug problem. An assessment could motivate and/or enable them to consider positive action.

SUGGESTED APPROACH
C : *How may I help you?*

The patient may complain only of depression, anxiety, or some other problem.

C : *What do you think might have caused these problems?*

If the patient does not come to the point:

C : *It seems you have had a tough time lately. How do you manage to cope?*

If the patent still does not come to the point, be more direct.

C : *Since you have come to this clinic, I presume you have a problem with drugs.*

Even if the patient makes a vague statement, encourage him.

C : *It is good that you have decided to seek help. It is never too late.*
What types of drugs do you use?

The patient may mention cannabis and alcohol only.

C : *What else do you use?*

P : Nothing much.

Ask slowly, giving him time to respond. Ask about cannabis, speed, ecstasy, cocaine, benzodiazepines, dihydrocodeine (DHC), heroin, morphine, methadone, co-codamol, Collis Brown, Gee's linctus, codeine linctus, painkillers etc.

If the patient admits using *opiates*:

C : *What did you start with?*

When did you start using it?

What did you try next?

How often do you use heroin?

How do you use it? [Smoking, snorting chasing, injecting]

How much heroin would you use on a typical day?

Does the amount you take vary from day to day?

How much would you use in a typical week?

On average, how much do you spend on them a week?

When did you start injecting [fixing] heroin?

How often do you inject?

Have you shared needles?

With whom have you shared needles?

Have you had any complications from injecting?

Have you ever been admitted to a hospital?

Have you had any tests for hepatitis or other infections?

Are you sexually active? Do you practise safe sex?

Ask similar questions as in 'heroin use' about other opiates also.

Tolerance, withdrawal symptoms and withdrawal relief

C : *What is the maximum you have had on a day?*

How much can you take without feeling drugged?

Has the dose you need for a kick gone up lately?

What would happen if you miss a dose? How do you manage it?

Do you experience withdrawal symptoms upon waking up?

Do you get body aches? stomach cramps? feeling nauseous and sick?

Do you feel anxious or tense?

Do you try to save some opiates to use on waking?

How long after waking up would you take your opiates?

Could you tell me if your drug use has been causing any problems for you?

Enquire about relationship problems, neglecting family, losing friends, financial problems, offending behaviour, convictions, problems at work, medical problems including hepatitis, depression, anxiety, suicidal behaviour etc.

C : *Have you tried to stop using drugs?*

> *Have you had any treatment in the past?*
>
> *How did it go?*
>
> *How long have you managed to go without any drugs?*

Compliment him for periods of abstinence.

C : *Have you ever attended Narcotics Anonymous?*

If yes, compliment him: *'It looks like you really tried hard.'*

C : *Why did things go wrong again?*

Insight and motivation

C : *Well, do you feel you have a problem with drugs?*

> *Are there any good things the drug does for you?*
>
> *Tell me if you find anything bad with using drugs.*
>
> *Do you feel that your opiate use has gone a bit out of control?*
>
> *Do people annoy you by asking you about your drug taking?*
>
> *Do you feel guilty about your drug habit?*
>
> *Do you worry about your opiate use?*
>
> *Do you wish you could stop?*
>
> *Why did you decide to come to us now?*
>
> *Are you due in court in the near future?*
>
> *Have you been in financial problems lately?*
>
> *Do you have any problems with your accommodation?*
>
> *What do you think about having a urine test for drugs?*
>
> *Have you had a blood test recently?*

Support systems

C : *Who do you live with? Do they also use drugs?*

> *How do you get on with your family?*
>
> *Is there anyone who is keen to see you clean?*
>
> *Would you like your family to be involved in the treatment?*

Background

The background history may reveal aetiological factors. Enquire about childhood, schooling, employment, relationships, offending behaviour unrelated to drugs, premorbid personality.

Summary and conclusion

C : *It appears you have a serious problem with drugs. The sooner we deal with it the better. It will not be easy, but we can try.*

> *What do you think? What do you want to do about it? What are your plans?*
>
> *I will give you some information on drug abuse problems and the help available. Feel free to discuss this with your family and friends. I hope to see you again next week.*

17 Explain lithium augmentation in depression

A. Jenaway

CONSTRUCT

The candidate demonstrates the ability to explain lithium augmentation of anti-depressant medication.

INSTRUCTIONS TO CANDIDATE

You are seeing a 35-year-old woman who suffers from recurrent major depression. Previous episodes have not responded to serotonin reuptake inhibitors but have responded to standard doses of tricyclic antidepressants within 6 weeks. She has now been on dothiepin 225 mg for 6 weeks but with only slight improvement and side effects of sedation, constipation and dry mouth. She is compliant with the treatment. Your consultant has proposed lithium augmentation. She knows a friend who was on lithium for bipolar affective disorder. You are asked to discuss lithium augmentation with her.

CHECKLIST

● Communication
● Explain the rationale
● Explain alternatives
● Describe the monitoring
● Describe side effects
● Describe toxic effects
● Explain the duration of treatment.

NB: Remember that lithium is used here to augment the antidepressant drug, not as a prophylactic agent.

SUGGESTED APPROACH:

Explain the purpose of the interview.

P : I thought lithium was only for manic depressives. Are you saying I'm manic depressive?

C : *No, I'm not saying that. You are right that lithium is used most often in the treatment of manic depressive illness, or better called bipolar affective disorder, where it acts as a mood stabiliser. It prevents mood swings into mania and into depression.*

Lithium can also be effective in preventing recurrences in patients with recurrent episodes of straightforward depression.

Another important use is where antidepressants alone have not been fully effective in getting the depression better. It helps about 50% of such people.

P : Is there anything else we could try?

C : *Well, we could try another antidepressant but you have not done well on the serotonin reuptake inhibitors in the past. It would mean withdrawing you from your current* *antidepressant and starting a new one. That could take some time and we would not know how you would respond. Another option would be cognitive behaviour therapy to look at the way you think and behave when you are depressed and see if you can change that, but that would also take some time and there is a waiting list. I think adding lithium is the best way forward at the moment. What do you think?*

P : It's quite toxic though isn't it?

C : *You are right in thinking it can be toxic but only in overdose or if the person is taking too high a dose. That is why we monitor the level in the blood to make sure you are taking the right amount. When we start lithium treatment, we start with a low dose and check the level after a week and adjust the dose as needed.*

P : How often will I have to have blood tests then?

C : *Before you start lithium you need a blood test to check your thyroid function and kidney function. We check your thyroid function because occasionally lithium can make the thyroid gland underactive and we want to check you don't have that problem already. We then check that every year to make sure it is still working normally. We check your kidney function because lithium is passed out of the body through the kidneys and we want to make sure there is no problem with your kidneys. We also check that every 6–12 months. You need to have lithium levels checked quite frequently when you are just starting on it, probably each week for a few weeks. After that, we need to check it only around every 4 or 6 months, except if you have had a change of dose or you are worried that the level might be too high.*

P : It still sounds a bit worrying to me. What side effects am I likely to get?

C : *Many people don't get any side effects as long as the dose is right for them. Some of the common side effects are a slight tremor in your hands, slight stomach upset, feeling a bit sick, a metallic taste in the mouth, drinking more and passing more urine than usual. Some people also gain weight on lithium.*

P : How will I know if the level is too high for me?

C : *If the level is too high you would notice a worsening of any side effects you already have or new ones coming. So you might have a marked tremor, diarrhoea and vomiting, unsteadiness in walking and clumsiness and slurred speech. If that occurs, you should stop taking your lithium and drink plenty of water. You need to have a blood test to check your level before you start the lithium again.*

P : How long would I have to keep taking it?

C : *That is difficult to be sure about. You need to continue on whatever medication gets you well for at least 6 months of being well before we review it and possibly start reducing it.*

18 | Assess a patient with early-onset dementia

A. Mitchell

CONSTRUCT
The candidate demonstrates the ability to take a history and examine a patient with suspected early-onset dementia

INSTRUCTIONS TO CANDIDATE
A 60-year-old single man, with no psychiatric history, but a history of a coronary artery bypass 5 years ago, presents to the outpatient clinic complaining of forget-fulness, getting lost in familiar places and word-finding difficulties. Perform a diagnostic assessment.

CHECKLIST
- History, mental state, cognitive function and physical examination
- Provide appropriate information and guidance.

SUGGESTED APPROACH

P : I have been concerned for some time that I have been having difficulty remembering names and speaking with friends. I hope I am not wasting your time.

C : *Not at all. I think we need to look at the problem in some detail. Could you tell me when you first noticed a problem and what were your main concerns?*

P : It began about a year ago when I had more and more trouble at work. I work as a maths teacher in a local secondary school, and I just kept making more mistakes. At first, I thought it was nothing, but then I noticed that I was forgetting people's names that I had known for years and then I couldn't get my words out properly. Before this, I was well, apart from my angina, but that improved with the bypass.

C : *Can you tell me about this and your heart bypass operation? Did you notice any changes after the operation?*

P : I have had angina for years and 5 years ago had a bypass. As far as I know everything went smoothly and I felt much better afterwards. My memory wasn't tested at the time, but didn't seem a problem. Do you think this is relevant?

C : *It is difficult to know at this stage, but memory problems are certainly a recognised complication of this procedure. Nevertheless, many other things could be involved. Do you mind if I run through some of these?*

History of cognitive complaints
Clarify the nature and severity of memory difficulties.

Problems in attention, concentration, planning, language, general knowledge – their effect on mood, social and occupational function and quality of life.

60 | **C :** *Have others noticed these?*

Aetiological screen

Family history of dementia, thyroid disease, depression or substance use.

Recent use of illicit or prescribed drugs.

Past history of affective disorder, psychosis, anxiety disorder.

Medical history, especially cardiovascular, cerebrovascular, endocrine, neurological.

Occupational risk factors.

Activities of daily living

Problems with advanced abilities: shopping, cooking and handling money.

Problems with basic abilities: self-care, eating, dressing and toileting.

Problems with social abilities: relationship, parenting, meeting friends.

Safety issues: driving, security, vulnerability, gardening, gas and electricity.

Compensatory strategies: notes, diary, mobile phone, reminders.

Social history

Enquire about work history and plans, home circumstances, level of informal and professional support, alcohol use, means of transport, changes in or relevance of hobbies and interests etc.

Neuropsychiatric and somatic symptoms

Apathy, agitation, disinhibition, irritability, anger.

Stereotyped rituals, behavioural problems.

Changes in eating, sleeping, energy/fatigue, sexual function, walking or senses.

Mood disorder (see 'Assess depression')

P : As I said, I do not feel depressed and don't have any of the symptoms you describe apart from the worry. Is there anything else you want to do while I am here?

Perform a mental state examination.

P : I am finding it difficult to answer all of your questions, but I can say that I have had problems in most aspects of memory and I avoid seeing friends in case I make an embarrassing mistake. Also, I have given up driving to work as it was getting too stressful – I get a lift now. Even at the moment, I am feeling on edge but I don't feel depressed. Why should I have trouble relaxing?

C : *That's a common problem in people with memory problems. It's easy to forget that life makes many demands on us day to day and we normally take these in our stride. However, when we have trouble with these it is natural either to avoid them, for example avoiding social engagements, or to ask others to help, for example getting a lift to work. In any case, being aware of these changes can be stressful. In some people, this progresses to a depression or anxiety state. It might be worth clarifying how much these worries have affected you, if that is okay.*

Now, I would like to test your memory, and do a physical examination.

Do a cognitive assessment (MMSE) and a focused physical examination.

- *General:* arousal, ventilation, tremor, sweating, pallor, clubbing, peripheral oedema
- *Vascular:* pulse, blood pressure, jugular venous pressure, signs of hyperlipidaemia, carotid bruit, examination of the precordium, heart sounds, basal crepitations
- *Neurological:* gait, speech and involuntary movements, cranial nerves, vision, ophthalmoscopy, changes in strength or sensation, balance, coordination, reflexes, primitive reflexes, ankle clonus, soft signs, e.g. sensory inattention, difficulty maintaining eye closure to command
- *Systemic:* liver, genitourinary system, dermatological examination.

P : Doctor, I hope you don't mind but I have looked up the causes of memory problems on the Internet. These are a bit complex. Can you clarify them for me?

C : *I hope you found a reputable site, as there is a lot of misinformation out there. Let's discuss memory problems in general and I can provide you with some further information if you wish. [Also see OSCE 20 'Explain Alzheimer's disease']*

Memory problems are very common particularly in later life and they do not always have a sinister cause. Indeed many causes are either reversible or treatable in some way. Some people are simply more aware of relatively subtle memory changes that occur as a normal part of aging. Not infrequently depression causes problems with attention or concentration. As you have probably discovered, when memory problems are more serious the explanation may be a medical condition affecting the brain. I have to emphasise that even in these cases some form of treatment is always available. I would like to do a simple blood test, which would rule out a wide range of conditions. Where memory problems are part of other complaints and last for many months some people call it dementia. However, I wouldn't call the condition you are suffering from dementia at this stage.

P : Thank you. That is very helpful. In summary, what do you think is going on?

C : *You have come to see me with several memory complaints that I take seriously and would like to continue to look into. It doesn't sound like depression is the cause but I would like to find out more about your heart operation from 5 years ago. With your permission, I would like to order your medical notes and speak with your GP. If a family member can come along to the next appointment, that would be helpful. Can I also ask if you would agree to a blood test, and a head scan? Some further memory tests would also help. I would like to see you again to review these. In the meantime I have some information sheets on memory loss that you might find useful, and I can give you some good Internet links if you like.*

REFERENCES

Nestor P, Hodges JR 2001 The clinical approach to assessing patients with early onset dementia. In Hodges JR (ed) Early-Onset Dementia: A Multidisciplinary Approach. Oxford University Press, Oxford, pp 23–47

Selnes OA, McKhann GM 2002 Cognitive changes after coronary artery bypass surgery. Curr Opin Psychiat 15: 285–290

Explain management of bipolar affective disorder

19

N. Hunt

CONSTRUCT

The candidate demonstrates the ability to establish a rapport with a patient and explain management and prognosis of bipolar affective disorder.

INSTRUCTIONS TO CANDIDATE

A 30-year-old married teacher has recently recovered from her first episode of severe mania and is at the end of her hospital stay. She is currently on lithium 800 mg. She wants to talk to you about the nature of the illness, its management and prognosis. She is planning to start a family.

CHECKLIST

- Explore knowledge and attitude
- Explain treatment and prognosis
- Encourage decision making
- Short-term and long-term planning
- Other sources of information.

SUGGESTED APPROACH

C : *I gather you want to talk about your illness and its treatment.*

P : That's right, I need to.

C : *I am pleased to hear that, as the more people know about their illnesses, the better. I presume that you would prefer to ask me questions, rather than me giving you a lecture. Please feel free to interrupt me.*

P : Can you tell me more about my diagnosis?

C : *As we have discussed previously, you have been suffering from a manic episode. Perhaps I should start by explaining a bit about mania. You are probably aware of the symptoms of mania. The good thing about mania is that it is usually a short-lived illness, which, with treatment, you would expect to recover from in a couple of months, as I think has happened with you. Do you know much about what can be expected for the future?*

P : I'd heard that it can come back and I need to take treatment for the rest of my life.

C : *Well, certainly part of that is true, that it can come back, although sometimes it comes back in a different form. People who have had a period of mania can experience another episode of mania but they can also suffer from the other side of the illness, which is depression.*

Have you ever had any problems with depression?

P : No I haven't, but my sister had a terrible bout of depression after she had her first child and ended up in hospital. It took her ages to recover.

C : *So you probably already know quite a lot about depression. It is because mania and depression seem to be linked in families and often occur in the same person that the illness is called manic depression. We also call it bipolar illness because there are the two poles of mania and depression.*

Do you know what the chances of having another episode of mania or depression are?

P : I've heard it's about 50/50.

C : *Well, if you are thinking about the chances of having either an episode of mania or depression in the next year or two that is about right. What is difficult if not impossible to know is which 50% you will be in. In the longer run most people do have another period of depression or mania. It is important that you and those who are close to you know this so that you can recognise it sooner rather than later.*

P : So should I carry on the treatment that I am on to prevent it coming back?

C : *You should certainly carry on the treatment that you are on at the moment for the next few months to make sure that you have put this episode of mania behind you.*

The more difficult and important question is whether you should take treatment in the longer term to prevent the illness coming back. Have you thought about that?

P : Well, I'm not getting any younger and I wanted to start a family, but I know that taking medicines when you are pregnant can affect the baby.

C : *That's true and particularly so for lithium. You should not get pregnant while you are taking lithium. Are you using contraceptives at the moment?*

P : Yes, my husband uses condoms.

C : *Fine. Perhaps we should talk a bit more about lithium. Have you heard anything about this treatment?*

P : Some people say it's terrible and knocks off your kidneys and your hormones, but I know that others swear by it.

C : *Well, let's start with the problems first. It's certainly true that you have to take lithium carefully because the level in the blood that's effective is only about half that which can make you very ill physically, including damaging your kidneys. Therefore, you need to have blood tests on a regular basis to make sure that the level in your blood is right. All of the lithium comes out through your kidneys and so you have to be sure that your kidneys are working properly, again by having regular blood tests. The other blood test that we regularly do is to check the thyroid gland, which produces hormones. This can be affected even if the lithium level is fine and so we need to keep a careful eye on this.*

P : Well, with all those problems why does anyone want to take it?

C : *People take it because it is the most effective way to prevent recurrence in manic depression. For about one in three people it makes a very major difference to their lives and successfully prevents them getting seriously ill again. For about another third it is helpful but not completely so. There are of course some people that it makes little difference to. One serious problem with it is that if you stop taking it suddenly then that can tip you into mania again. Had anyone told you that?*

P : Yes, they told me that on the ward and I can assure you that I don't want to go back to that again. I know that arrangements are being made for me to have regular blood tests.

C : *Even with the blood tests being done you need to be aware that if you are unwell physically, particularly with vomiting and diarrhoea, that could be a sign that the level is too high and you need to get some medical advice quickly. We also need to make sure that you have a good information leaflet about lithium.*

Anyway, coming back to where we go from here with your treatment: are you happy to continue the treatment over the next few months to make sure that you have recovered well?

P : Yes, I am happy with that but I do not want to take it in the longer run, as I want to have a baby.

C : *Did you know that having a baby could trigger another episode of mania?*

P : No. How common is that?

C : *The chances are that about one in every three women who have suffered from manic depression will have a relapse after childbirth. I will be happy to discuss that with you, and if you wish, with your husband also.*

I hope that we have touched on some of the important issues for you and given you some things to think about regarding your longer-term treatment. We've agreed that you will continue the treatment as it is for the moment and that it will need to be reviewed with your specialist in out-patients. You also know some of the important aspects of lithium treatment. I would encourage you to find out more about manic depression, perhaps by joining an organisation like the Manic Depression Fellowship, so that when you come to make the longer-term decision about preventative treatment you are happy that you have made the right decision. You might also find that talking to others with similar problems can help you to look at other aspects of your life that can have an impact on manic depression, for example how much you drink or if you take other drugs.

20 | Explain Alzheimer's disease

A. Tarbuck

CONSTRUCT

The candidate demonstrates the ability to establish a rapport with the relative of a patient diagnosed as suffering from Alzheimer's disease. The candidate explains the nature, aetiology, signs and symptoms, treatment and likely outcomes in a manner that the relative can understand.

INSTRUCTIONS TO CANDIDATE

Mrs Jones is the daughter of a 79-year-old man (Mr Smith) who was seen recently in the 'memory clinic'. He lives with his 81-year-old wife. His general practitioner referred him with a 1-year history of progressive memory problems. Following assessment in the clinic including blood tests, a CT scan and neuropsychological assessment, the diagnosis of early Alzheimer's disease was made. Mrs Jones has made an appointment to see you to discuss aspects of her father's condition. Before this appointment you have obtained Mr Smith's permission to discuss his condition with his daughter.

CHECKLIST

- Empathic approach
- Use non-medical language
- Allow the relative to express her concerns
- Be alert to her concerns for her parents
- Explain common signs and symptoms of Alzheimer's disease
- Discuss potential problems that could occur
- Discuss prognosis
- Explain treatments
- Explain practical help available, e.g. social services care, financial assistance
- Offer hope but avoid false reassurance.

SUGGESTED APPROACH

C : *What can I do for you, Mrs Jones?*

R : Thank you for seeing me, doctor. Can you tell me exactly what is wrong with my father, please?

C : *As you know, your mother and family doctor have had concerns about your father's memory. We saw him in the specialist memory disorders clinic. We also found that he has definite memory difficulties and we carried out some tests to clarify the cause. Our results suggest that his memory problems are most likely to be due to a condition called Alzheimer's disease.*

R : Couldn't this just be due to my father's age? After all, he is 79!

C : *There is often some decline in the ability to learn new information as people get older, but these changes are usually quite mild and subtle. Unfortunately the changes we have found in your father are more severe than this and indicate that he does have a medical condition that is causing his problems.*

R : What tests have you done and what did they show?

C : *We interviewed your parents to obtain a clear history of his problems and the way in which they developed. We also asked questions about his mood to make sure he was not depressed, because depression can cause memory problems.*

We did a physical examination, which did not reveal any signs of physical illnesses that could cause his memory difficulties.

We did some blood tests to exclude conditions such as problems with his thyroid gland or certain vitamin deficiencies that can sometimes cause memory loss; these were all normal.

A clinical psychologist assessed his memory and other brain functions in more detail. Her tests showed that your father does have clear problems with remembering things, and also that he has some difficulties with organising information and making judgements.

Finally, we did a CT brain scan. This is a special X-ray of his brain. It showed that there has been some shrinkage of his brain tissue, but no evidence of strokes or anything like a brain tumour.

R : What is Alzheimer's disease?

C : *Everyone loses brain cells as they get older. In people with Alzheimer's disease, this process is more severe and rapid than in normal ageing. The parts of the brain that deal with memory are usually affected first. Someone with this condition becomes increasingly forgetful and has great difficulty learning new information, although memories for things from very many years ago tend to be preserved much better. This means that sufferers often lose things around the house and ask the same questions again and again. Later on, other parts of the brain are affected and people may develop problems with their speech or with undertaking practical tasks like preparing meals or getting washed and dressed.*

R : Does that mean he is definitely going to get worse?

C : *Unfortunately, it is a progressive condition. Although your father has been started on a drug that may slow the deterioration in memory function, it is not a cure and ultimately I'm afraid that he will deteriorate.*

R : Is he going to become violent towards my mother?

C : *Violence is not an inevitable consequence of Alzheimer's disease. Unfortunately, aggressive outbursts do occur in between 18% and 65% of patients. However, they are more usually verbal rather than physical and tend to occur later on in the illness. Aggression is more common in patients who have a poor relationship with the person caring for them, and in people who have a history of being aggressive earlier in life. Neither of these is true in the case of your father.*

R : How long has he got to live?

C : *I'm afraid that is an extremely difficult question to answer. Some people have survived for up to 16 years after being diagnosed. Most studies have shown people to live for*

5–6 years after being diagnosed. However, we are now making the diagnosis earlier on in the disease process, as in your father's case, and so it is likely that these figures may be an underestimate. However, these are only average figures and it really is not possible to make firm predictions in individual patients. Your father's illness is relatively mild at present and he is in good physical health for his age.

R : How will my mother be able to cope with looking after him on her own? You do realise that she is 81 herself?

C : *We know that your mother will need help and support. We have already started organising this. As well as coming to the 'memory clinic' to monitor his response to the drug treatment, we have invited your mother to join the relatives' support group. We have also arranged for one of our community nurses to visit your parents at their home. She will be keeping an eye on the home situation, and both you and your mother will be able to contact her for advice. She will work with our social worker to ensure that your parents receive all the benefits to which they are entitled and that they are offered appropriate practical help.*

R : What sort of help can Social Services offer?

C : *If your father needs help with personal care, such as washing or dressing, then a home carer can visit to assist him. Social Services can also arrange for him to attend a luncheon club or day centre to provide him with some stimulation and company and to allow your mother to have a break. They are also often able to provide short stays of 1–2 weeks in a residential home to provide relatives a longer period of respite. Should your mother eventually feel that she cannot manage to care for your father at home then Social Services can help to organise permanent care in a suitable residential or nursing home.*

R : Where can I obtain more information about Alzheimer's disease?

C : *The Alzheimer's Society is extremely helpful. They produce various books and leaflets, and they have a good web site if you have access to the Internet. Your father's community mental health nurse has a lot of experience in helping people with Alzheimer's disease and she will be very happy to talk with you. I would also be very happy to answer any further questions you may have in the future.*

R : Thank you for your time, doctor.

Elicit history of eating disorder

21

D. Bermingham

CONSTRUCT

The candidate demonstrates the ability to form a rapport with a young woman and to elicit an eating disorder history. The candidate rules out a depressive illness. The candidate discusses the diagnosis, possible complications and treatment.

INSTRUCTIONS TO CANDIDATE

You are asked to see a 20-year-old shop assistant who has insulin-dependent diabetes mellitus. The GP was concerned about her diabetes control and the patient admitted to omitting her insulin in order to lose weight. She came for the appointment reluctantly. Elicit history of eating disorder.

CHECKLIST

- Be courteous and supportive. Avoid confrontation
- Presenting complaint
- Current eating pattern.

Common features

- Extreme concerns about and disturbed perception of weight and shape
- Body image disturbance, disparagement, loathing
- Fear of fatness and weight gain
- Determined pursuit of thinness and weight loss.

Distinguishing features

Anorexia

- Body weight below 85% of that expected
- Denial of the seriousness of current low body weight
- Amenorrhoea.

Bulimia

- Near-normal body weight
- Binge eating with a sense of lack of control
- Compensatory measures
- Self-evaluation unduly influenced by body shape and weight
- Preoccupation with food.

- Co-morbidity and suicide risk
- Explain diagnosis and management.

SUGGESTED APPROACH
Ask about the presenting complaints.

Get a clear picture of the current eating pattern.

Start with what the patient ate the previous day.

Preoccupation with food
Ask about preoccupation with food, fear of losing control, overeating and periods of craving for food.

Binge eating
Ask her to describe a typical binge.

Enquire about the frequency and a sense of lack of control.

Look for triggers for binges – dysphoria, interpersonal stress, starvation, feelings related to body weight and shape.

Are they planned or impulsive?

How do the binges end?

How does she feel and what does she do afterwards?

Measures to counteract the fattening effects of food
Self-induced vomiting, restricting fluids, exercising, use of laxatives, purgatives, appetite suppressants and thyroid derivatives, dieting, calorie limits, avoiding particular types of foods, skipping meals, periods of starvation, chewing and spitting.

In diabetes – manipulation of the insulin dose.

Weight history
Current weight, ideal weight and changes in weight.

Fear of gaining weight.

Frequency of weighing.

Body image disturbance
Extreme concerns about and disturbed perception of weight and shape.

Body image disturbance, disparagement and loathing.

Self-evaluation unduly influenced by body shape and weight.

Fear of fatness and weight gain.

Determined pursuit of thinness and weight loss.

How often would she measure parts of the body or look in the mirror?

Associated behaviours
Cooking rituals, cooking for others, avoiding eating in front of others, stealing food, shoplifting.

Menstrual history

Age of menarche, regularity of periods, periods of amenorrhoea, last periods.

History

Onset, duration, change in pattern, i.e. from anorexia to bulimia.

Aetiology

Predisposing, precipitating and maintaining factors.

Premorbid personality

Consider obsessive, anxious, borderline personality traits.

Effects

How is the eating disorder affecting life in general, studies or work, relationship with parents, social life, relationships, libido etc.?

Discuss physical and other complications.

Co-morbidity

Rule out depression, alcohol and drug misuse, personality difficulties, OCD and physical problems.

Mental state

Look for specific psychopathology, depression, obsessions and suicide risk.

Explain diagnosis

In a non-judgemental and supportive manner.

Explain treatment

The aim of treatment is to help the patient regain control over eating.

Physical examination, blood tests, ECG and dietary advice.

Psychological treatments, e.g. CBT and interpersonal psychotherapy.

The role of antidepressant drugs.

Suggest keeping a diary of eating until review next week.

Offer information leaflet including a list of useful books.

22 Explain antidementia drugs

J. S. Rubinsztein

CONSTRUCT

The candidate demonstrates the ability to establish a rapport with the carer of a patient with Alzheimer's disease and explain antidementia drugs.

INSTRUCTIONS TO CANDIDATE

Explain antidementia drugs to the wife of a patient with Alzheimer's disease.

CHECKLIST

- Empathy
- Types of drugs
- Mechanism of action
- Contraindications
- Side effects
- Benefits
- Monitoring
- Avoid false reassurance
- Offer support.

SUGGESTED APPROACH

C : *I am sorry that your husband has been diagnosed as having Alzheimer's disease. I gather you want to discuss possible drug treatments for him.*

P : Yes, but I have heard the treatment is expensive. Will we have to pay for this treatment?

C : *No, these drugs are now available on the NHS. Shall I explain to you about these drugs? Please feel free to interrupt me.*

P : All right.

C : *Recently some new drugs have been made available for the treatment of mild to moderately severe Alzheimer's disease. These include donepezil, rivastigmine and galantamine. More drugs are on the way e.g. memantine. Your husband may be suitable for one of these drugs. Shall we discuss further the use of donepezil, the one I would like to consider prescribing?*

P : How will this drug help him?

C : *It will not cure him. It may help to stabilise the illness or improve it for a while. It may help his memory. More often carers see general improvements in behaviour or mood. Some patients with Alzheimer's disease seem to take more interest in life and are able to do more for themselves after starting this drug.*

P : How does the drug work?

C : *In Alzheimer's disease, one of the chemicals in the brain called acetylcholine is in short supply. The drugs act by increasing the brain levels of acetylcholine.*

P : How do we go about starting the drug?

C : *We have to find out if the drug suits your husband. Has he ever had stomach ulcers, asthma, chronic shortness of breath or chronic coughing [COAD]?*

P : No.

C : *Does he suffer from severe heart, kidney or liver problems?*

P : No. He is very well except for his memory problems.

C : *Does he take any drugs?*

P : None. Why did you ask?

C : *One has to be very careful to avoid interactions with certain drugs. They include erythromycin, fluoxetine (enzyme inhibitors), rifampicin, phenytoin, carbamazepine (enzyme inducers) and drugs for arrhythmias such as digoxin.*

P : Are there any side effects?

C : *Yes, but these are not usually troublesome.*

The most common problem is feeling nauseous or a bit sick in the beginning. Therefore we recommend taking the drug with food. If your husband feels very sick or if he vomits, then he would not be suitable for this drug. If he develops any other side effects then we may have to reconsider whether it is worth continuing this drug.

P : How is the treatment given?

C : *We will start with one tablet of 5 mg of donepezil (Aricept) once a day. I will need to re-evaluate this dose in about 5 weeks. I shall ask a nurse to see your husband after about 2 weeks of treatment to make sure that he is not having side effects.*

P : How long would he stay on the drug for?

C : *Initially we will see if at 3 months your husband has shown any benefits from this drug. If not, we may take him off the drug. If he does show improvement then we will need to review him approximately every 6 months to see if it is worthwhile continuing the treatment. In some patients, if we stop the drug because there has not been any apparent benefit they may deteriorate rapidly and we may have to consider reintroducing the drug.*

Is there anything else you would like to ask me?

P : I am not sure what to do.

C : *Yes, I understand. There has been too much on your plate lately. I think you need some time to think things through. I will give you some written information on the management of Alzheimer's disease. It has details about Age Concern, the Alzheimer's Disease Society and other support groups and self-help groups. I would like you to go through it and discuss it with your family, friends and your doctor. I will see you again next week to make a decision about the drugs and also discuss the other supports that can be arranged. You are welcome to come with a relative or a friend.*

23 | Assess challenging behaviour

M. Woodbury-Smith

CONSTRUCT

The candidate demonstrates the ability to establish a rapport with an adult with a mild learning disability and his carer, communicate effectively and elicit the nature and possible causes of challenging behaviour.

INSTRUCTIONS TO CANDIDATE

A GP has referred a 43-year-old man with Down's syndrome and mild learning disability who has become increasingly difficult to manage in the residential home where he lives. Assess the patient and interview the carer to identify the nature of the behavioural problems and the aetiological and associated factors.

CHECKLIST

- Presenting problem
- Previous functioning
- Environmental causes: bereavement, conflict with staff and other residents, change in staff or staffing levels, change in his routine, people moving into or leaving the residential home, issues related to family, e.g. contact with family
- Neuropsychiatric causes: anxiety, depression, epilepsy, Alzheimer's disease
- Other physical causes: infections, pain, hypothyroidism
- Get permission from the patient to communicate with the carer
- Leading questions may be necessary
- Confirm the answers with carer as you go along.
- * Indicate questions to the carer.

SUGGESTED APPROACH

C : *Hello, my name is ____ . I am a doctor. I am here to help you. Your doctor has asked me to see you because he/she is worried about you. I would like to talk to you and your carer about this. Is that okay?*

The presenting problem

C : *I understand that there have been some problems lately. What happened?*

Have you been doing anything that you don't usually do?

How have you been getting on with people?

How well have you been eating lately?

Have you been participating in your usual activities at the home?

Have you been losing your temper?

Have you been shouting at people?

Have you been smashing furniture?

What else have you been doing that you don't usually do?

I would like to ask your carer about what has been going on. Is that okay?

Ask the carer how the patient's behaviour has been different.

Previous functioning

C : *Do you like living at the home?*

What about the others who live there?

Do you like the staff at the home?

How do you get on with them?

Do you ever argue with them?

Tell me what sorts of things you get up to during the day and evenings.

What are your favourite activities?

Which ones do you not like doing?

Do you go to a day centre?

How are things there?

Have you ever done anything like this before?

Ask the carer about the patient's behaviour before the current problems.

Environmental causes

C : *Did something upset you just before things went a bit wrong for you?*

Can you tell me why you have been getting upset lately?

Has anyone of the staff left the home recently?

Have there been any new staff?

Has one of your mates left the home recently?

Did anyone new come to live at the home?

Can you tell me about your family?

Cross-check with the carer.

Mood

C : *Do you worry about things?*

What sort of things do you worry about?

What do you feel like when you are worried?

Do you feel your heart beating fast?

Do you feel shaky or sweaty?

How do you feel in your mood?

If he does not understand, draw happy and sad faces on a scale and ask him to indicate where he thinks he is on this scale.

C : *Why is your mood not so good?*

Have you cried lately?

When is the worst part of the day?

Do you still enjoy doing your favourite things?

How long does it take before you fall asleep?

What time do you wake up compared with others?

Are you the first or the last to wake up?

What about eating? Do you still like your food?

Have your clothes become too tight or loose lately?

How do you feel in your energy?

How do you see the future?

Do you at times feel that you do not want to be alive?

Have you thought about harming yourself?

What do you think you might do?

Ask the carer appropriate questions to confirm the patient's report, e.g. mood, crying spells, diurnal variation, interests, activities, sleep, appetite, weight, energy, communication of hopelessness and suicidal thoughts.

Other psychiatric symptoms

C : *Do you have any unusual experiences that you can't explain?*

What about frightening things happening to you?

Do you hear voices when you think you are alone?

Can you tell me about them?

Are you worried about people being out to get you or trying to harm you?

If any of the answers suggest, enquire more specifically for psychotic symptoms.

Ask the carer if there has been any evidence of such symptoms.

Skills and memory

C : *What are you like at remembering things?*

Is it all right if I ask your carer about some of the things you do around the house?

* Can you tell me a bit about his self-care and daily living skills?

* Does he wash and dress himself independently?

* Does he need prompting, supervision or support?

* Does he feed independently?

* Can he find his way around the house?

* Does he recognise familiar staff?

* Does he know his way around the neighbourhood?

* Has there been any change in these skills?

* Has there been any change in any other skills, for example verbal skills?

Physical causes

C : *Do you have any pain anywhere?*

Do you have a cough?

Do you have a sore throat?

* Is he on any regular medication?

* Does he seem to be in pain at all?

* *Does he look to be in pain when he walks?*
* *Does he have epilepsy?*
* *Has he had any blackouts, fits or funny turns recently?*
* *When was the last time his thyroid function was checked?*

24 | Elicit history of panic attacks

M. F. Okhai

CONSTRUCT

The candidate demonstrates the ability to elicit the history, symptoms, severity and complications of panic attacks.

INSTRUCTIONS TO CANDIDATE

A 26-year-old married woman with two children aged 1 and 3 years is referred by her GP because of her fear that she is going mad. Make a diagnosis based on history taking.

CHECKLIST

- Clarify presenting complaints and history
- Aetiology: precipitating factors, stresses
- Progression of symptoms: safety behaviours and avoidance, anticipatory fear, development of agoraphobia and other phobias, disturbed sleep and nocturnal attacks
- Comorbidity: depression, OCD, somatization
- Effect on family and friends
- Risk of self-harm
- Substance misuse: alcohol, drugs, stimulants, nicotine – as aetiology & self-medication
- Medical history
- Family history
- Recapitulate
- Explain treatment.

SUGGESTED APPROACH

Presenting complaints and history

C : *I understand that your GP has referred you because you are afraid that you may be going mad?*

P : Yes I've been having these horrible attacks.

C : *Can you tell me what happens when you have these attacks?*

P : I am terrified that something terrible is going to happen. I used to think that I was having a heart attack but my doctor tells me my heart is fine.

C : *Why did you think that you were having a heart attack?*

P : Because my heart beats like the clappers.

C : *Does anything else happen when you have these attacks?*

P : I can't breathe, I feel sick, sweat, shake, and when it's really bad I get pins and needles, and a strange feeling like I'm not real – that's sort of hard to explain.

C : *What else do you fear might happen?*

Enquire about fears of heart disease, going insane, humiliation in public etc.

C : *How long does an attack last?*

P : Seems like for ages but I know they can't have been longer than 5–10 minutes.

C : *How are you in between attacks?*

P : Perfect, except worrying when I'm going to get the next one and how I'm going to cope.

Onset, possible precipitants

C : *When did you have your first attack?*
What were you doing at the time?
What do you think brought the attack on?
What was going on in your life at the time?
Was everything going well?

Progression of symptoms, family influences

C : *How often have you been getting these attacks?*
Have they been getting more frequent?
Where are you and what are you doing when they start?
Are they more likely to occur in any particular situation?
They are terrifying. How else have they been affecting you?
Would you do anything to avoid them?
Would you avoid situations that might cause the attacks?
Can you describe them, please?
Are these attacks causing any difficulties between you and your husband?
How are these attacks affecting the rest of your family?

Risk of self-harm

C : *Have you got to a stage where your attacks have been so bad that you wanted to do something drastic?*
Have you thought it all too much and wanted to just end it all?

Co-morbidity

Consider depression, OCD.

Substance use

Consider both causative agents and attempts at self-medication.

Enquire about caffeine, nicotine, alcohol and drugs.

Associated medical problems

Enquire about medical problems, investigations and treatment.

Consider irritable bowel syndrome, mitral valve prolapse, thyroid function tests, ECG.

Family history

C : *Does anyone or has anyone else in your family had these attacks or any similar problems?*

Recapitulation

C : *Well, from what you have told me I can assure you that you are not going mad. You are having panic attacks. The name given to the number and types of attacks you are having is panic disorder. A panic attack happens when your body, mistakenly sets off what is called the fight-or-flight response. Would you like me to explain that?*

When we are in danger the body prepares us either to fight the danger or to run away or flee. The fast heartbeat and the heavy breathing are part of the body gearing us for fighting or fleeing. However, in the case of panic attacks there is no obvious danger. Not being able to see danger while the body is all geared up for it is frightening, and this fear makes all the symptoms even worse. Often panic attacks seem to start 'out of the blue', but there is usually added stress around the time of the first attack. In your case it may have been the worry over your husband's job and the stress of looking after your two young children. Once you had your first attack your body was sort of looking out for the next one, so it may have been something quite minor that set the second one off and then the cycle got worse and worse.

Explain treatment

C : *Fortunately, we have good ways of treating panic attacks. We can treat you with medication but the attacks may start up again when we try to get you off the medication. Psychological methods, which means teaching you to use techniques and strategies to get rid of your panic attacks, are much more effective in the long run.*

Differentiate depression from dementia

B. A. Lawlor

CONSTRUCT

The candidate demonstrates the ability to elicit the clinical features of depression and dementia and in particular the features that will best distinguish them in a sensitive and empathic manner.

INSTRUCTIONS TO CANDIDATE

An elderly lady has been referred to you for assessment. She is worried that she has dementia. You are asked to decide whether this patient is suffering from dementia or depression. Please take a history and perform a Mental State Examination as part of your assessment.

CHECKLIST

- Empathy
- Establish rapport
- Symptoms of depression
- Symptoms of dementia
- Past psychiatric history
- Past medical history
- Medications
- Family history
- Personal history, especially, aetiological factors, life events, alcohol, smoking etc.
- Mental State Examination, especially suicide risk and cognitive function
- Feedback.

SUGGESTED APPROACH

C : *Good morning. My name is ____ . As you know, your doctor asked me to see you in relation to your concerns about your memory. I would like to start from the beginning. Can you tell me how long you have been feeling unwell?*

P : I haven't been myself for about a year. I seem to be on edge all the time and have lost my confidence. I can never remember anything, where I left things, what people have said to me. It is very frustrating.

C : *How did it all begin?*

P : Just over a year ago I lost my husband. Things just haven't been right since then.

C : *I am sorry to hear that. How did he die?*

P : Suddenly, after a heart attack.

C : *How did you cope at that time?*

Enquire briefly about grief reaction.

Enquire systematically about *depressive symptoms*, suicide risk, anxiety symptoms and any psychotic symptoms. If psychotic symptoms are present, determine if they are mood congruent or not. Determine if the depressive symptoms have persisted since they began, and if they are getting worse.

If there was any period of improvement in depression, did the forgetfulness also improve?

Enquire about the onset and extent of the *cognitive symptoms*, i.e. memory, language problems, disorientation etc.

In particular, try to establish which came first: depressive symptoms or memory complaints.

Ask open-ended questions. For example:

C : *You mentioned at the beginning that you are worried about forgetfulness. Tell me more about that, please.*

P : I forget where I leave things, what I wanted to say and the details of recent conversations. Once I was supposed to drop my grandchild home on the way to the shops, and I arrived at the shops with her. That really worried me.

C : *I am sure that was distressing for you. How long have you noticed this for?*

P : I have been aware of it for about 6 months now.

C : *Did you have any concerns about your memory before your husband died?*

P : No doctor, I was a different woman then, always out and about, and it never entered my head.

C : *How do the memory difficulties affect you, for example, about the house?*
Have you made mistakes with bills or shopping?
Are you finding it hard to keep up with housework?

P : I might forget where I have left something, or what I wanted in the shop, but nothing important yet. I have less interest in the house, but I push myself to do it. It keeps my mind off things, and so far I am keeping up.

The candidate should then gently enquire about other cognitive symptoms, word-finding problems, temporal and spatial disorientation. It is important to use open questions in this situation, so as not to be suggestive to a depressed patient. Look for functional decline by asking about changes in the past year.

After a detailed assessment of the presenting symptoms, focus on the onset, progression and severity of depressive symptoms versus cognitive symptoms. Then look into the other parts of the history.

Past psychiatric history: A past history of depression suggests a current diagnosis of depression is more likely.

Ask about past medical history and medication, including any treatment that the GP has prescribed for her current symptoms.

Family history: Family history of depression is more suggestive of a diagnosis of depression, and a family history of dementia is more suggestive of that.

Relevant issues in personal history, predisposing, precipitating factors, or perpetuating factors, life events, alcohol, smoking etc.

After completing the history, perform a *cognitive assessment*. Introduce this in a sensitive manner. During the history taking the candidate should have some opinion of the patient's long-term and perhaps short-term memory. The MMSE would be a suitable cognitive assessment. A depressed patient is likely to give 'I don't know' answers, and will need gentle encouragement. Persist with them to give you an answer.

Patients with early dementia will give some incorrect answers. Again, the examiner should be encouraging, minimising the impact of wrong answers and praising them when they get one right. Both patients with depression and those with dementia may do poorly on the tests of memory. However, with depression this is due to problems with attention and concentration, which will be evident from other aspects of the assessment, whereas with dementia it is more likely to be a problem with memory processing per se. Moreover, a normal Clock Drawing Test would be more suggestive of depression than dementia.

Feedback

The patient might ask how they did and whether they are losing their memory or not. The candidate should acknowledge the memory symptoms that they are having. You should explain that there are a number of causes of symptoms of poor memory, including depressive illnesses, and that you believe they are suffering from depression at present. Explain how depression can result in memory difficulties. Inform them that in order to rule out other causes of memory difficulties you would like to do further tests, including blood tests and a brain scan. The most important thing, however, is to treat the depression and then to retest memory.

26 Elicit borderline personality traits

C. Denman

CONSTRUCT

The candidate demonstrates the ability to establish a rapport with a patient with borderline personality disorder and to elicit the characteristic personality traits.

INSTRUCTIONS TO CANDIDATE

A 27-year-old woman presents in A & E with slashes to her wrists. She has a long history of repeated overdoses and deliberate self-harm. While the casualty officer was suturing the slashes, she became angry and abusive towards him. She picked up a scalpel and threatened to cut herself. You are asked to elicit symptoms of borderline personality disorder and explain the diagnosis to the patient.

CHECKLIST

- Identity disturbance
- Intense and unstable relationships
- Efforts to avoid abandonment
- Recurrent suicidal behaviour
- Chronic feelings of emptiness
- Impulsivity
- Inappropriate intense anger
- Affective instability
- Transient stress-related paranoid and dissociative symptoms
- Explain diagnosis.

SUGGESTED APPROACH

Identity disturbance

Enquire about the patient's goals/plans in work/friendships/romantic life.

C : *Looking back over your life, do you feel that your goals often change?*
Has your tendency to change plans made life difficult for you in any way?

Unstable and intense emotional relationships

Take a longitudinal relationship history. Ask also about relationships with carers – professional and otherwise.

C : *How have your relationships worked out for you?*
Could you explain?

Efforts to avoid abandonment

C : *How often do you feel abandoned/left to cope on your own?*
What happens (how do you react) when you feel this way?

Has this interfered with your life and made things bad for you?

Recurrent suicidal behaviour

In this case, there is a confirmed history of repeated self-harm behaviour.

Chronic feelings of emptiness

C : *Do you often feel as though you are empty inside? As though life is meaningless?*
How often do you feel bored?
Do you feel bored even when you are doing something you ought to enjoy?
Has this feeling led you to do things you regret or to harm your life?

Impulsivity

C : *Do you ever do things impulsively and then regret them? How often?*

Ask further about spending habits, sexual risk taking, substance abuse, reckless driving, binge eating etc. (Do not include DSH.)

Affective instability

Enquire about moods and feelings, how often they change and how long the low moods last. This should be hours or rarely a few days but not persistent low mood.

Inappropriate intense anger or difficulty controlling anger

C : *Do you think you have a problem with your temper?*
Could you elaborate on it, please?
Have you got into fights?

Ask about forensic history.

Transient stress-related paranoid and dissociative symptoms

For paranoid symptoms, see 'Elicit delusions'.

C : *Do you ever feel unreal or cut off, like a zombie?*
Is this feeling one you can control and end or is it one you can't control?
Have you ever had periods in your day/week you can't account for properly?
Have people ever told you that you were behaving strangely for a while but you were not aware of it?

Co-morbidity

Depression: Look for sustained bouts of low mood with biological symptoms.

Anxiety: Look for persistent increased vigilance and classic symptoms of anxiety.

Distinguish panic attacks from dissociative symptoms.

Substance abuse, eating disorders, psychosis, complex PTSD.

Past history

Early abuse, physical, emotional, sexual – at home and at school.

Neglectful, emotionally inconsistent and unpredictable care giving.

Difficulties at school suggestive of impulse control problems.

Adolescence: Distinguish from adolescent experimentation.

Adult life: Relationship, social and work history.

Emotional history

Associated with receiving care, e.g. hospital admissions, previous psychotherapy.

C : *How did you feel about the carers? Ideal? Rejecting? Dismissive?*

Current functioning

Work/education, social, intimate relationships/sex life.

Is she content in these areas?

Does she have plans for the future? Are these achievable?

Risk of harm to self

Although patients with BPD make many threats of harm to self/others compared with the number of acts they commit, their risk of completed suicide is very high (8%).

Risk of harm to others

History: Aggressive outbursts, forensic history, association with alcohol/drug use.

Current: Recent/active threat, evidence of preparation, e.g. stalking, harassing, trial run, carrying a weapon, current stated intent.

Future: Likely opportunities, provoking factors.

Explain diagnosis

C : *It is likely that the main reason for your problems is that you have something called borderline personality disorder. Is this something other people have suggested?*

P : Staff on the ward said I was a PD and they wanted to discharge me.

C : *Yes, this diagnosis sometimes makes people feel as though they are being accused of being a bad person. It actually means that you may have been born with, and/or your early experiences have left you with, problems in calming yourself down, in relating to people and in feeling confident about who you are and how you feel. I expect that often you may feel a very strong mood or wish that seems to come on for no reason and then change into another one without explanation.*

P : When I feel angry or depressed I cut myself and people say I am manipulative.

C : *People with personality disorders are often called manipulative when they do things over which they have little control. In addition, you have probably found that you have made many decisions in your life which were impulsive and which turned out badly for you. All these things are part of having borderline personality disorder.*

P : Having a personality disorder means there is no cure for me, doesn't it?

C : *People often feel that there is no hope for them. In fact, there are now quite hopeful treatments for personality disorders. Even if you have always been someone whose feelings and thoughts can be all over the place, you can learn ways of limiting the damage that the impulsive acts and decisions do to your life plans. The main thing is that all the treatments mean lots of hard work from you and they can be emotionally quite painful. It is much more like exercise classes than like taking a pill.*

Explain long-term psychoanalytic psychotherapy

27

M. Robertson

CONSTRUCT

The candidate explains the nature of long-term psychoanalytic psychotherapy to a patient with borderline personality disorder.

INSTRUCTIONS TO CANDIDATE

You are an SHO in the psychotherapy department. One of the consultant psychiatrists has referred a young woman with borderline personality disorder to your department for long-term psychoanalytic psychotherapy. Your consultant has asked you to explain the nature of this treatment to this patient.

CHECKLIST

- Clarify patient's understanding of referral
- Elicit patient's expectations of psychotherapy
- Establish previous psychotherapy experiences and difficulties
- Explain therapeutic relationship and boundaries
- Explain transference and resistance
- Set ground rules of therapeutic contract.

SUGGESTED APPROACH

C : *I understand that your consultant psychiatrist has referred you for long-term psychotherapy and that you want to know more about it.*

P : So I believe.

C : *Can I start by asking what you already know about the treatment?*

P : I know that it will take 1 to 2 years of one to two visits per week and that I stand to benefit a lot, but I don't know what it involves.

C : *Perhaps you could tell me about the treatments you had before?*

P : I have been on antidepressant medication for years.

C : *Do you feel that it has helped?*

P : Yes, I think so, but I still seem to have a lot of difficulties in my relationships and I still feel very bad about myself at times.

C : *Have you had any psychological or talking treatments?*

P : Well, my consultant psychiatrist used to spend a little bit of time with me talking about how things were in my life.

C : *Could you tell me a little bit more about that?*

P : She felt it helped, but really it did not do much for me. She didn't seem to have a lot of time for me and I also thought she didn't really understand me very well.

C : *Did you find you were developing very strong responses to her?*

P : What do you mean, 'strong responses'?

C : *Did you find yourself becoming angry with her or did you find it was difficult to cope in between your sessions?*

P : Well, I did find that despite the fact it made me angry, I really needed to get to each session. I would often be there a half an hour before the appointment. Sometimes I would drive around the clinic for an hour before that.

C : *Did you ever talk about this with your psychiatrist?*

P : Not really.

C : *Perhaps we could talk a little bit about long-term psychotherapy.*

P : All right then.

C : *Well, as you are probably aware, psychotherapy refers to a number of different talking treatments. These treatments can vary from being fairly brief, often one or two sessions, but can often go on for 2 to 3 years. It is very much a case of tailoring the treatment to the person's needs.*

Your consultant referring you for long-term treatment perhaps suggests that your needs are more complex and that it will take time for you to settle into the treatment to obtain the full benefit.

P : Really?

C : *Yes. There is one thing basic to all the different types of psychotherapy, which is the formation of a therapeutic relationship.*

P : What do you mean, 'relationship'?

C : *Well, it is the bond of attachment that forms between the patient and therapist, and it is very much like any other relationship.*

P : You mean like a friendship?

C : *Well, not quite a friendship. You see, your therapist is bound by professional ethics. Your therapist will be taking the position of being a helping professional. His or her relationship with you needs to be guided by a set of rules. This would include things such as how much of his or her own details is disclosed in treatment sessions, the arrangements you have for contact out of hours, and in private psychotherapy, rules about payment etc.*

P : I have heard about patients and therapists who have relationships.

C : *Well, this is the very reason why there needs to be a set of rules to govern the way in which the therapeutic relationship occurs.*

P : Oh.

C : *Because of your needs and your vulnerability, it is important that you and your therapist understand the need for what we call boundaries.*

P : Boundaries?

C : *Yes, boundaries, which really refers to the set of rules governing therapeutic relationships.*

P : I see.

C : *The other thing to be aware of with longer-term psychotherapy is that they focus on the mechanics of the relationship.*

P : Mechanics?

C : *Yes, you have described having certain responses to your consultant when she was treating you. In a longer-term treatment, it is important that you form a stable and helping therapeutic relationship with your therapist. It is also helpful to look at the nature of your responses to your therapist as these can often help in understanding the experiences you have in life.*

P : You mean the unconscious?

C : *Exactly. In psychotherapy, the responses to therapists are called 'transference'. Transference refers to the unconsciously determined responses that you have to your therapist. For example, you becoming angry or frustrated in your previous treatment might be important as it can tell us a little bit about your expectations and also the unconscious aspects of your behaviours in relationships.*

P : I see.

C : *You also need to be aware that some of the frustrations in psychotherapy come from another process called 'resistance'.*

P : Resistance?

C : *Yes, resistance refers to the process of the patient in psychotherapy attempting to maintain his or her own status quo. In many cases, psychotherapy tries to engender change in people's way of thinking, feeling and acting as well as their experience of relationships. People are the way they are because of their life experience and the other things that go to make up their personality. If you try to change these in psychotherapy, you will no doubt encounter this resistance. This is a normal part of treatment and is very much in the same league as the other process of transference we talked about.*

Do you have any questions so far?

P : No, I think that is fine, thank you.

C : *Good. Another thing we have to discuss is a 'contract' in therapy.*

P : You mean like a business contract?

C : *Well, sort of. A psychotherapy contract tries to set out the rules for the way in which the therapy is going to occur. We will need to talk about things such as how many sessions per week we have. How long will these sessions be? What should happen if there are problems after hours? What are acceptable behaviours during the therapy sessions? The rules for missed sessions or lateness. We will talk about that in some depth in our next session.*

Would you like to ask me any questions before we finish?

P : No, thank you.

C : *I will give you some written material with more detailed information about the various aspects of psychotherapy. If you have any further queries, I will be happy to see you again.*

28 | Elicit passivity experiences

P. J. Mathai

CONSTRUCT
The candidate demonstrates the ability to establish a rapport with a patient presenting with psychotic symptoms and to elicit passivity experiences.

INSTRUCTIONS TO CANDIDATE
A GP has referred a young man with psychotic symptoms. Elicit passivity experiences, if any.

CHECKLIST
● Introduce the topic tactfully
● Thought insertion
● Thought withdrawal
● Thought broadcast
● Thoughts being read
● Passivity of affect
● Passivity of impulse
● Passivity of volition
● Somatic passivity
● Clarify the details: attribution, distress, ego alien and the degree of conviction
● Conclusion.

SUGGESTED APPROACH
C : *I would like to ask you some questions that we ask everyone who comes to us. Some of them may appear a bit strange. Tell me if you have any difficulty with any of them, or if you are not sure what they mean. Is that all right with you?*

Screening questions
C : *I gather that you have been under a lot of stress lately. When under stress people can have certain unusual experiences. Has anything unusual or strange been happening to you?*

Have things happened that you find difficult to explain?

Has there been any difficulty with your thoughts, feelings, actions or bodily sensations?

Thought alienation
This includes thought insertion, withdrawal, broadcast and thoughts being read.

C : *Are you able to think clearly?*

Have you had any difficulty with your thinking recently?

Has there been any interference with your thoughts?

Do you feel that you are always in control of your thoughts?

Is there anything like telepathy or hypnosis going on?

Thought insertion
C : *Usually whatever one thinks are his own thoughts. Has it been the case with you too?*
Does someone put their thoughts into your mind?
Do you have thoughts which are not your own, but coming from elsewhere?
How do you know that they are not your own thoughts?
Where do they come from?
How do you think they get into your mind?
Can you explain them, please?

Thought withdrawal
C : *Do your thoughts sometimes stop quite unexpectedly, leaving none in your mind?*
Do you sometimes feel that your thoughts are taken away from your mind?
Would that leave your mind empty or blank?
Can you give an example, please?
Can you explain how it happens?

Thought broadcast and diffusion
C : *Do you sometimes hear your own thoughts spoken aloud in your head, so that someone standing near you might hear them?*
Do your thoughts seem to be somehow public, not private to yourself, so that others can know what you are thinking?
Do others know what is in your mind, as if your thoughts are being broadcast?
How do you explain it?

Thoughts being read
C : *Can people read your thoughts?*
How do you know that?
How would you explain that?

The last question on passivity of thought
C : *Is there any other kind of interference with your thoughts?*

Other passivity experiences
C : *Are you always in control of what you feel and do?*
Is there someone or something trying to control you?
Is there someone or something forcing you to say or do things?
Is there any kind of outside control over your feelings, impulses or actions?
Do you feel under the control of some force other than yourself?
… As though you are a robot or a zombie without a will of your own?
… As though you are being possessed by someone or something?

Passivity of affect
C : *Is there someone or something trying to change the way you feel in yourself?*

Does this force or person sometimes force its feelings on to you against your will?

Passivity of impulse

C : *Have your intentions been replaced with those of others?*

Passivity of volition

C : *Do you feel that your will has been replaced by that of some force outside of yourself?*

Can you describe that, please?

Somatic passivity

C : *Is there something like X-rays or radio waves affecting your body?*

Do you think that someone produces strange experiences on your body?

Do you think that someone plays on your body?

Do you sometimes feel like a robot or a puppet controlled by someone and without a will of your own?

Clarification

C : *Who do you think is doing these things?*

How do they do that?

Why do they do so?

How often does it happen?

Is there anything that would make these experiences more likely?

Do they happen against your will?

Can you resist them?

How do these things affect you?

How distressing are they?

How do you react to such experiences?

How do you cope with this experience?

Have you ever wondered if these things are really happening or if your imagination is playing tricks on you?

Is there anything else that I have not asked you about or you would like to talk about?

Conclusion

C : *Thank you very much for explaining these things so clearly. We call them passivity experiences. I appreciate that they are very unpleasant experiences. I hope that you will get better soon.*

Resuscitation

B. Smith

CONSTRUCT

The candidate demonstrates the ability to perform cardiopulmonary resuscitation (CPR).

INSTRUCTIONS TO CANDIDATE

A 50-year-old man has collapsed on the psychiatric ward in a general hospital. You are called to attend. Demonstrate how you would assess the patient and perform emergency cardiopulmonary resuscitation if required.

CHECKLIST

- Call for help
- Ensure safety
- Check responsiveness (shake, shout)
- Open airway (head tilt, chin lift). Jaw thrust if cervical spine injury suspected
- Check breathing (look, listen, feel).
- If breathing, put patient in recovery position
- If not breathing and help has not arrived, leave patient and get help (remember – think defibrillator)
- Deliver two effective breaths
- Assess circulation for 10 seconds (not breathing, not moving and no carotid pulse)
- If circulation is present, continue rescue breathing and check for signs of circulation every minute
- If circulation is not present, start chest compression.

SUGGESTED APPROACH

Call for help

As you approach the patient, check the environment for dangers, and immediately shout for help.

If the collapsed patient is an adult, the most likely cause of a sudden collapse is ventricular fibrillation (VF) and the only proven therapy is defibrillation. For each 1-minute delay in defibrillation there is a 7–10% reduction in the chances of a successful outcome. Therefore the quicker the defibrillator arrives, the better the outcome. Hence, call for the cardiac arrest team or ambulance before starting resuscitation.

There is very little benefit in performing CPR for 1 minute prior to getting help as in most cases this merely serves to delay defibrillation. The only possible exception is for children as VF is unlikely to be a cause of their arrest. Try to take the child with you when going to call for help – if possible performing basic life support (BLS) en route.

Safety

Ensure your safety and that of the patient. Tell the examiner that you would not endanger your life or the lives of others while attempting to resuscitate the casualty.

Responsiveness

Ask loudly 'Are you all right?' Shake his shoulders.

The patient does not respond.

Airway

Tilt his head back gently by pressing on his forehead with your hand. With your fingertips under the victim's chin, tilt the chin to open the airway. Remove any obstructions in the mouth.

Breathing

Check for breathing for 10 seconds.

Put your ear to his mouth and check for breathing.

Look at his chest for movement.

Check for carotid pulse simultaneously (optional).

If breathing, put the patient in the recovery position.

If not breathing, go and get help.

Rescue breathing

If not breathing and help has been summoned, remove any obstructions from the patient's mouth, e.g. dislodged dentures. Leave well-fitting dentures in place.

Ensure that the airway is still open, using head tilt and chin lift.

Close his nostrils by pinching with the thumb and index finger of your hand on his forehead.

Open his mouth slightly, but maintain chin lift.

Place your lips around his. Blow into his mouth slowly and steadily for 2 seconds, watching for his chest to rise.

Take your mouth away from the patient and watch for his chest to fall as the air is expired.

Give a second breath. You can have up to five attempts at delivering the two effective breaths.

Check Circulation

If not already done, check carotid pulse for 10 seconds while looking for other signs of life, including movement, swallowing or breathing

Chest compression

If there is no evidence of a circulation, start chest compressions immediately.

Position yourself vertically above the victim's chest.

Place the heel of your one hand over the middle of the lower half of the sternum. Place the other hand on top with the fingers interlocked. Keep your arms straight. Press down on the sternum to depress it 4–5 cm downwards. Make sure that your fingers do not press on the ribs.

Release the pressure, but don't take your hands off the sternum. Repeat this approximately 15 times within 10 seconds, with equal duration for compression and release. Aim for a rate of 100 compressions per minute.

After 15 compressions, tilt the head, lift the chin and give two more effective breaths.

Return without delay to resume chest compressions.

Continue chest compressions and breaths at a ratio of 15 to 2.

Reassess the ABC's only if the patient visibly improves.

Continue until help arrives, the patient shows signs of life, you become exhausted or the examiner asks you to stop.

NB: Competence in BLS is essential for all health professionals.

This is best achieved by supervised practice with a suitable manikin. CPR cannot be practised on live human volunteers.

30 | Assess frontal lobe function

M. Moran

CONSTRUCT

The candidate demonstrates the ability to assess frontal lobe functions, including performing simple bedside tests in a sensitive and empathic manner.

INSTRUCTIONS TO CANDIDATE

Assess frontal lobe function in this man.

CHECKLIST

- Empathy, rapport and patience
- Initiation
- Planning
- Perseveration, motor or verbal
- Sequencing/motor control
- Abstraction
- Cognitive flexibility
- Verbal fluency
- Category fluency
- Primitive reflexes.

SUGGESTED APPROACH

C : *My name is ____ . Your doctor has asked me to see you today as he is concerned that you have not been yourself lately. I want to do some quick tests of memory and concentration with you. Firstly, if you could tell me about yourself and how you have been feeling?*

Allow the patient time to speak freely, observe for overfamiliarity, disinhibition, irritability, distractibility, apathy, lack of emotional concern and perseveration.

P : I feel fine. There is nothing wrong with me. My wife says I am not myself, that I am too friendly with strangers, and that I want to have sex all the time. I do not see anything wrong with that.

C : *Do you have any complaints yourself?*

P : No I feel great. How about you, doctor, you look a bit pale. Do you mind if I call you by your first name?

C : *I am fine, Mr ____ . Now let's do some of these tests I was talking about.*

Some of the following tests can be used to assess frontal lobe function. Many of these tests are qualitative, and hence it is important to document exactly what difficulties the individual has with them.

Tests for motor control, and the ability to initiate a task and to follow a sequence of instructions

These tests may also illustrate perseveration. It will not be necessary to complete all the following tests.

C : *Put your left hand on top of your head and close your eyes.*

Move quickly onto next task. The patient should not hold the posture during the next task.

C : *Well done. Now when I tap once under the table, you tap twice on the table and when I tap twice you tap once.*

I would like you to say some numbers and letters for me like this, 1A, 2B, 3 … What should come next? Now you try starting with number 1. Keep going until I say stop.

Using a pen and paper, ask the patient:

C : *Can you please continue with the following design?*

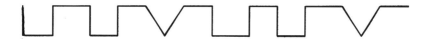

Finger–nose–finger task

Candidate holds up his right index finger.

C : *Touch my finger.*

Leaving finger in place, the candidate says:

C : *Now touch your nose.*

The patient should stop touching your finger and touch his nose with the same hand.

Go/No-Go tasks

C : *When I touch my nose, you raise your finger like this.*

Candidate raises right finger.

C : *When I raise my finger you touch your nose like this.*

Candidate touches nose with right index finger.

Have patient repeat the instructions if possible.

Candidate begins task. Leave finger in place while awaiting patient response.

Luria hand sequence

C : *Can you do this?*

Candidate demonstrates a sequence of hand positions: from a slap, to a fist to a cutting position.

C : *Now follow me, and keep doing this until I say stop.*

Candidate stops, and the patient should have three successful cycles without error after the candidate stops.

Abstract reasoning

C : *What do I mean when I say 'a stitch in time saves nine'?*

Or

C : *What do I mean when I say 'a rolling stone gathers no moss'?*

Or ask the patient to describe the similarities and differences between an apple and an orange.

Fluency

C : *Name all the words you can in 60 seconds beginning with the letter D.*
Well done, now with the letter A.

Or

C : *Now could you name all the animals you can think of in 60 seconds?*
Well done. Now all the fruit and vegetables.

The patient should get 15 plus depending on age and educational level.

Cognitive estimates

C : *How tall is an average Irish woman?*
What is the best paid job in Britain?
What is the largest object normally found in a house?

Primitive reflexes

Grasp reflex: Grasping of the contralateral hand when stroking the palm from the radial to the ulnar side.

Pout reflex: Pouting of the lips, elicited by either stroking down the filtrum or by gently tapping on a spatula placed over the lips.

Palmomental reflex: A wince on stroking the ipsilateral thenar eminence.

C : *Thank you for your cooperation and well done.*

Fundoscopy

A. J. Vivian

CONSTRUCT
The candidate demonstrates the ability to examine the fundi and describe the findings.

INSTRUCTIONS TO CANDIDATE
Do a fundoscopic examination of a 50-year-old man complaining of headaches and describe your findings and interpretation to the examiner.

CHECKLIST AND SUGGESTED APPROACH
Explain that

- You have to look into the back of his eyes using this light.
- We have to do it with the light in the room switched off.
- The light can be uncomfortable.
- You will have to come so close to the patient that your face may touch his.

Get the patient's permission.

If the patient is a female and the doctor is a male, ask for a chaperone.

Ensure that the ophthalmoscope is working. Turn it on. Check the light.

Ask the patient to remove his glasses and look at an object at a distance and at eye level and to blink and breath normally.

Either keep your own glasses/lenses on or remove them and dial up the appropriate lens for your refractive error; –lenses for myopia and +lenses for hypermetropia.

Stand or sit on the side to be examined at 1 metre from the patient and with your eyes level with the patient's.

Use your right eye to examine the patient's right eye and your left eye to examine the left eye.

If you have difficulty using your non-dominant eye, you can examine the patient from above, so that the patient can continue to fix on a distant object.

Switch on the ophthalmoscope. Check the patient's lens for opacities. Set the lens at 0. Look through the aperture and shine the ophthalmoscope light at the patient's pupil, angling it slightly towards the nose. Dial up the high + red numbers. Normally there will be a red reflex due to light reflecting from the back of the retina. An absent red reflex may be due to cataract or other opacities.

Keep your other eye open.

Consider your eye and the ophthalmoscope functioning as a single unit. Bring your eye slowly towards the patient's eye until you are as close as possible without touching the eye lashes.

The back of the patient's eye should be in focus. If not, adjust the lens, keeping close to the patient. For long-sighted patients, try a convex/positive lens in increasing strength. Use a negative/concave lens for short-sighted patients.

When the retina is in focus, follow a blood vessel to the optic disc. The optic disc is slightly pink, with sharp borders and a central cup.

Look at the four arteries and the accompanying veins, especially where they cross each other.

Look for pallor, swelling, new vessel formation, exudates and haemorrhages.

Locate any abnormality as though the fundus is a clock with the disc at the centre. The diameter of the disc (1.5 mm) is used as the unit of measurement. For example, hard exudates at 6, 7 and 12 o'clock, 2–3 disc diameters from the disc.

Look at the macula by asking the person to look directly at the light and using a narrow beam.

Examine both eyes.

Report findings to the patient or to the examiner, in case of a manikin.

Thank the patient.

NB:
Do not annoy the patient with your foul breath.

Do not annoy the patient with prolonged dazzling.

You may get a patient, a manikin or a photograph. In the latter two cases, explain to the examiner what you would tell the patient.

The best ways to train yourself are to attend the ophthalmology–diabetic clinic and to include ophthalmoscopy as part of the routine physical examination.

1. Normal left fundus

The main components of the fundus are the macula, the optic nerve (optic disc), the nasal and temporal retinal vessel arcades and the peripheral retina.

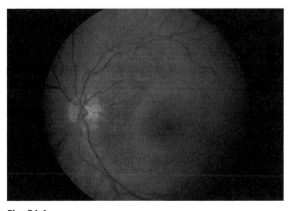

Fig. 31.1

The macula is the central area of the retina surrounded by the temporal arcade of vessels and is used for fine, detailed vision.

The optic disc is situated on the nasal side of the macular area and carries the nerve fibres from the eye to the brain. Because there is no retina overlying the optic disc, it creates a blind spot in the visual field.

Because the optic nerve is offset on the nasal side of the fundus, the superior and inferior blood vessel arcades are larger on the temporal side surrounding the macula than on the nasal side.

The fovea is the pink central point of the retina in the middle of the macula, and is responsible for the most detailed vision (such as reading).

2. Normal right fundus

The disc is nasal to the macular area.

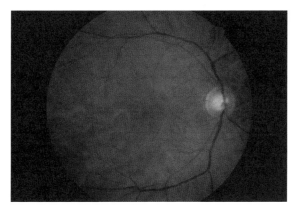

Fig. 31.2

3. Normal pigmented (Asian) left fundus

The fundus is much less pink in Asian individuals.

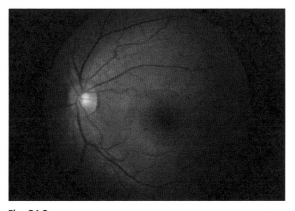

Fig. 31.3

4. Papilloedema

Papilloedema is a swollen optic disc caused by raised intracranial pressure.

The disc margins are indistinct.

The retinal arteries and veins of the disc are not clear.

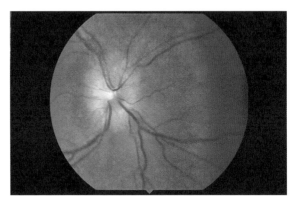

Fig. 31.4

5. Optic atrophy

Optic atrophy is the late result of damage to the optic nerve. There are many causes.

The disc is very pale and featureless

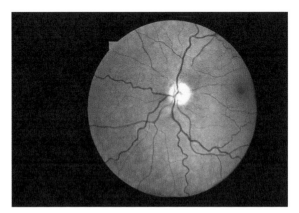

Fig. 31.5

6. Cupped left optic disc

Normal optic discs are composed of a small, pale central cup surrounded by a pink rim. The cup should occupy less than 50% of the total diameter of the optic disc.

If the optic disc cup occupies greater than 50% of the disc diameter it is suggestive of glaucoma.

This photo shows the optic discs in a pigmented fundus. The left optic disc cup occupies almost 80% of the disc diameter. This is abnormal and typical of the optic disc seen in glaucoma. The right disc is normal.

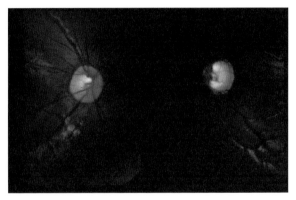

Fig. 31.6

7. Afro-Caribbean fundus

The fundus in Afro-Caribbean individuals is much darker than Caucasians or Asians.

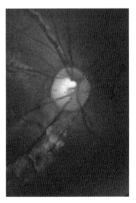

Fig. 31.7

8: Central retinal vein occlusion (left eye)

Thrombosis of the central retinal vein causes widespread haemorrhages through-out the retina. It occurs most commonly in association with hypertension.

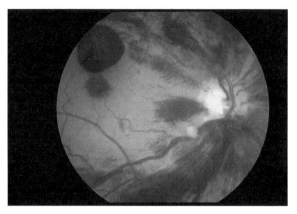

Fig. 31.8

There are multiple flame-shaped haemorrhages in the nerve fibre layer.

There are also some large blot haemorrhages.

9. Branch retinal vein occlusion (left eye)

If thrombosis occurs in one of the smaller retinal veins, only a small area of the retina is affected.

There are flame-shaped haemorrhages in the superior macular area.

Within the area of haemorrhage there is a cotton wool spot.

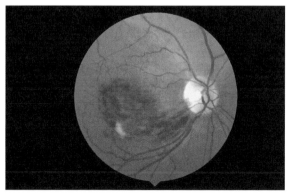

Fig. 31.9

10. Background diabetic retinopathy (right eye)

Background diabetic retinopathy is characterised by dot and blot haemorrhages throughout the fundus. In addition there may be exudates.

There are multiple exudates in the macular area.

There are scattered 'dot and blot' haemorrhages throughout the fundus.

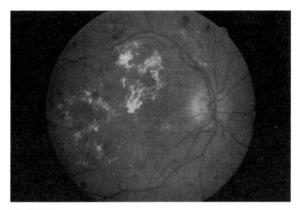

Fig. 31.10

11. Proliferative diabetic retinopathy with new disc vessels

Advanced diabetic retinopathy is more common in insulin-dependent diabetics. It is characterised by the development of fine 'new vessels' either at the disc or along the vascular arcades.

There is a network of fine new vessels around the disc.

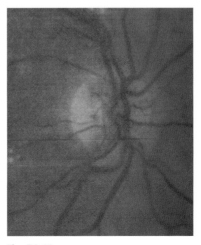

Fig. 31.11

12. Drusen at the macula

Fine yellow dots surround the fovea in the macular area. These are called drusen and are an early sign of age-related macular degeneration (ARMD).

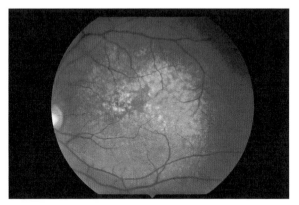

Fig. 31.12

13. Hypertensive retinopathy

Early hypertensive retinopathy is characterised by narrowing of the retinal veins where they are crossed by the retinal arterioles (not shown in this patient).

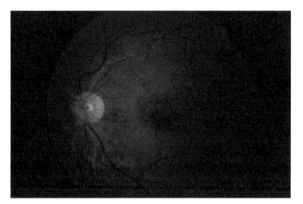

Fig. 31.13

More advanced hypertensive retinopathy is characterised by the development of small flame-shaped haemorrhages, blotchy haemorrhages and exudates often centred around the macula.

Explain cannabis and psychosis

32

R. Rao

CONSTRUCT

The candidate demonstrates the ability to establish a rapport and communicate the relation between cannabis use and psychiatric illness.

INSTRUCTIONS TO CANDIDATE

One of your in-patients is a 20-year-old man who has just recovered from an acute psychotic episode, possibly a cannabis-induced psychosis. He had persecutory delusions and auditory hallucinations. While on home leave from the ward he smoked cannabis again and had a worsening of his psychotic symptoms. The nurses tell you that he does not think that cannabis is the cause of his illness because most of his mates smoke cannabis and are well. Discuss the relation between cannabis and mental illness with him.

CHECKLIST

- Empathy
- Motivational interviewing style
- Acknowledge that cannabis use is common and may have relaxing effects
- Explain the link between cannabis and psychiatric disorders
- Explain vulnerability
- Explain the impact of cannabis use on prognosis
- Enquire about other drugs
- Stress the patient's responsibility.

SUGGESTED APPROACH

Try to use the same words as the patient, such as 'pot' or 'weed'.

C : *I would like to discuss your illness and its treatment with you. Is that all right with you?*

Can you tell me why you had to come to the hospital?

Can you tell me how it all started?

The patient may be evasive.

C : *I am sure you remember that you have been hearing voices, feeling that people were against you and you were very scared. Do you remember what happened then?*

P : I became better. I stopped hearing voices and feeling paranoid.

C : *You are correct. You became better and everyone was so pleased. We had discussed the reason why you became ill. Do you remember what made you so ill?*

P : You lot told me that it was because I have been smoking pot, but I did not use any strong stuff ...

C : *Yes. We had all agreed that cannabis was the reason for you becoming unwell. Then you told us that you had given it up for good. We suggested that you contacted the Drug Advisory Services. What happened then?*

P : I wanted to be discharged. You agreed to let me go on leave.

C : *You are correct. How did your leave go?*

What did you do while on leave?

Did you meet your mates?

Do they know what your problem is? I mean, why you are in the hospital?

Did you feel tempted to try cannabis?

Did you try?

How much did you smoke?

Did you use any other drugs?

What effect did it have?

Did it cause any problems?

Can you explain it a bit more, please?

If the patient denies any problems:

C : *I gather that the voices came back on your return from leave. Am I right?*

What would you attribute this to?

How do you think cannabis is affecting you?

If the patient continues to be defensive:

C : *As we have discussed many times before, it appears that cannabis caused your illness and other problems. You got better when you stayed off cannabis for many days and had some medication. It seems that just a few puffs made you unwell again. If I again suggest that cannabis makes you very unwell, what would you say?*

P : But it makes me feel relaxed and most of my mates take it as well.

C : *Yes. Cannabis can make some people relaxed. That is the reason why it is so popular. I appreciate that many of your mates smoke cannabis and they enjoy it without any problems. I know it is difficult for you not to join them.*

However, cannabis causes severe problems for some people. People can get stoned with cannabis. Some become suspicious and paranoid. Some others get what we call a cannabis-induced psychosis when they become out of touch with reality, start hearing voices and become paranoid and convinced that people are trying to harm them. This is very much like schizophrenia, except that it usually improves with stopping cannabis and taking medication. However, it can come back when people use cannabis again. I am afraid this is what happens to you.

Tell me what you think.

P : Why am I different from my mates?

C : *Cannabis has different effects on different people. It is difficult to predict how different individuals react to this drug. Some are more susceptible to the bad effects of cannabis than others. Unfortunately, you are one of them.*

P : How would I know if I am susceptible?

C : *In your case, it looks as though there is a strong link between smoking cannabis and feeling paranoid and hearing voices. You got better when you were on the ward and not smoking cannabis. Then the few puffs you have had while you were on leave also appear to have made your voices worse.*

P : How can cannabis cause these symptoms?

C : *Cannabis contains a chemical called THC, which affects certain chemicals in the brain. This produces symptoms similar to that of a major mental illness like schizophrenia. However, if the symptoms are solely due to cannabis they will usually go away a week or two after you stop using cannabis. The symptoms usually come back if you use cannabis again.*

P : You are trying to control me.

C : *We are only trying to tell you how to remain well. The choice is yours.*

P : Would I be able to smoke some cannabis if I take my medication regularly?

C : *I am afraid that cannabis will cause problems even if you take medication regularly. Research has shown that people who became unwell because of using cannabis have a high chance of having more relapses and hospital admissions if they use it again.*

P : Even if I become ill again, you will be able to sort me out. Won't you?

C : *That is true. However, each time you become unwell and develop symptoms like those you had recently, your brain gets damaged more and more. The improvement will be best the first time you become unwell. You may not make as good a recovery on future occasions. Moreover, recent research has shown that heavy use of cannabis for long periods can increase the chances of schizophrenia by up to four times.*

P : But everyone, including researchers, say cannabis is a safe drug.

C : *First, there are no safe drugs. The studies which showed that cannabis was relatively safe were done many years ago. The cannabis that is available these days is up to 30 times more powerful or has 30 times more THC than what was available in the 1960s and 1970s.*

P : I have been smoking cannabis for ages. All my mates smoke cannabis. It is not easy for me to stop just like that.

C : *I fully agree with you. It will not be easy. However, stopping cannabis is the only way you can remain well and stay out of the hospital. Our Drug Advisory Service will be able to give you counselling and support. They can teach you ways of coping without using cannabis. I will give you their telephone number.*

P : Why don't you refer me to them?

C : *We would like you to take the first step. They will be keen on you contacting them directly rather than us referring you. We would like you to be in control of your life.*

Interpret ECG

D. MacDougall

CONSTRUCT

The candidate demonstrates the ability to interpret ECG.

CHECKLIST

- Rate
  Divide 300 by the number of large squares between each QRS complex.
- Rhythm
  This can be regular or irregular. To assess rhythm, lay a card along an ECG and mark the position of three successive R waves. Slide the card back and forth to check that all the intervals are the same.
- Axis – The normal axis lies between −30° and +90°.
  If the QRS complexes in leads I and II are predominantly positive, the axis is normal.
  Left axis deviation exists if lead I is positive, and both leads II and aVF are negative.
  Right axis deviation occurs if lead I is negative, and leads II and aVF are positive.
- P wave – This is caused by depolarisation of the atria. Normal height and width are less than 2.5 mm and 0.11 s, respectively, in lead II.
- PR interval – The range is 0.12–0.20 s, or three to five small squares.
- QRS complex represents ventricular depolarisation. Its duration is less than 0.12 s, or less than three small squares. If more than 0.12 s, a conduction defect is likely.
- Q waves – These are pathological if they are more than 25% of the height of the following R wave, and more than 0.04 s wide (one small square).
- ST segment is normally isoelectric (flat). It can become elevated acutely in myocardial infarction or pericarditis. ST depression occurs in several conditions, including myocardial ischaemia and left ventricular hypertrophy.
- T wave represents ventricular repolarisation. T wave inversion in lead I, II, or V4-6 is usually abnormal. Peaked T waves can occur in ↑K^+. T wave can be flattened in ↓ K^+.
- QT interval – The interval between the beginning of the QRS complex and the end of the T wave. It varies with heart rate, and so must be corrected: the QTc, or corrected QT interval. To calculate the QTc, divide the QT interval by the square root of the preceding R–R interval (the latter is the interval between the R waves of two successive QRS complexes). It should be less than 0.42 s.

ECG 1

A 28-year-old woman is admitted with a severe depressive disorder. On the ward, she complains of palpitations and tingling in her fingers. Hence an ECG was done.

Describe the ECG.

What do you do next?

Suggested approach

The ECG shows normal sinus rhythm at a rate of 60/min.

The axis is normal.

The P waves are of normal morphology.

The PR interval is about 0.12 s (three small squares or just over half a large square), which is normal.

The QRS complexes, ST segments and T waves are normal.

There are no abnormalities. This is a normal ECG.

Tingling in fingers suggests hyperventilation. I will reassure the patient that her ECG is normal. I will explore anxiety symptoms and suggest anxiety management training.

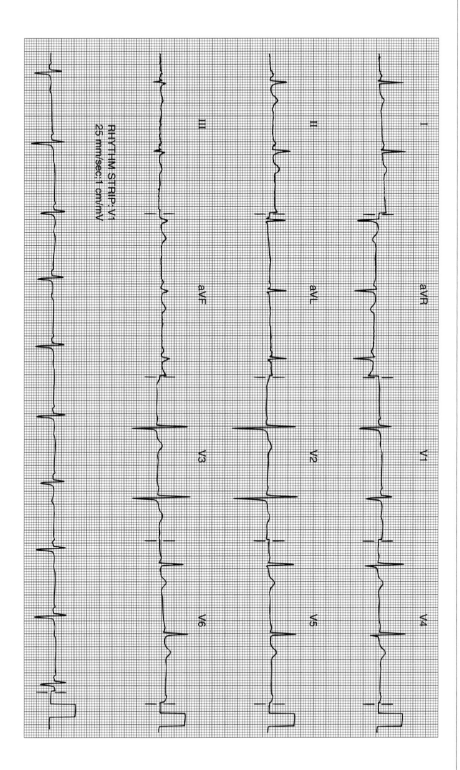

RHYTHM STRIP: V1
25 mm/sec;1 cm/mV

ECG 2

A 58-year-old diabetic woman on your ward complains of central chest tightness and sweating.

What does the ECG show?

What do you do next?

Suggested approach

The ECG shows a sinus tachycardia of 114/min.

The axis is normal.

P wave morphology is normal.

The PR interval is 0.2 s (five small squares), which is just the upper limit of normal.

The QRS complexes are normal.

There is ST segment depression in the anteroseptal leads (V2–V5).

There is T wave flattening in the anterolateral leads (1, aVL, V4–V6).

This is very suggestive of acute anterior myocardial ischaemia.

I will take a full history and do physical examination.

I will contact the medical registrar immediately.

If available, I will give oxygen and attach her to a cardiac monitor until medical help arrives.

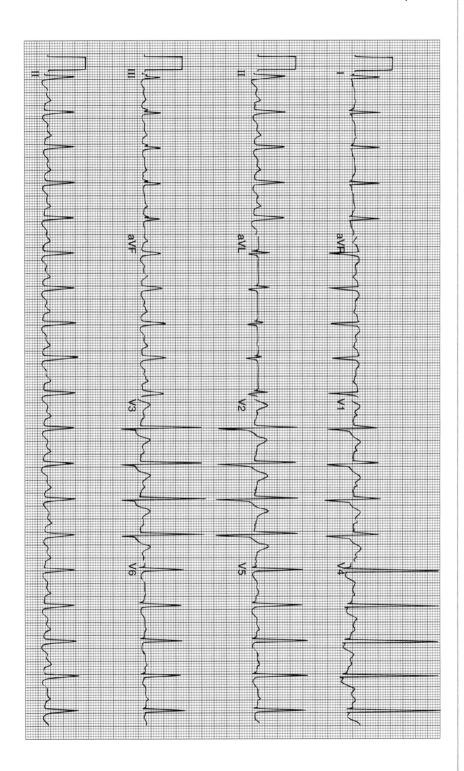

ECG 3

A 53-year-old man on your ward complains of central chest tightness and difficulty in breathing.

What does the ECG show?

What do you do next?

Suggested approach

ECG shows sinus rhythm at a rate of 66/min.

The axis is normal.

The P waves are of normal morphology.

The PR interval is 0.16 (four small squares), which is normal.

The QRS complexes are normal.

There is ST segment elevation in the lateral leads (I, aVL, V5, V6) and reciprocal ST depression in the inferior leads (II, III, aVF).

The T waves are peaked (hyperacute) in the anterior leads (V2–V4) and inverted in the inferior leads (II, III, aVF).

This is highly suggestive of an acute anterolateral myocardial infarction.

I will take a full history and do a physical examination.

I will contact the medical registrar immediately.

If available, I will give the patient oxygen and attach him to a cardiac monitor until medical help arrives.

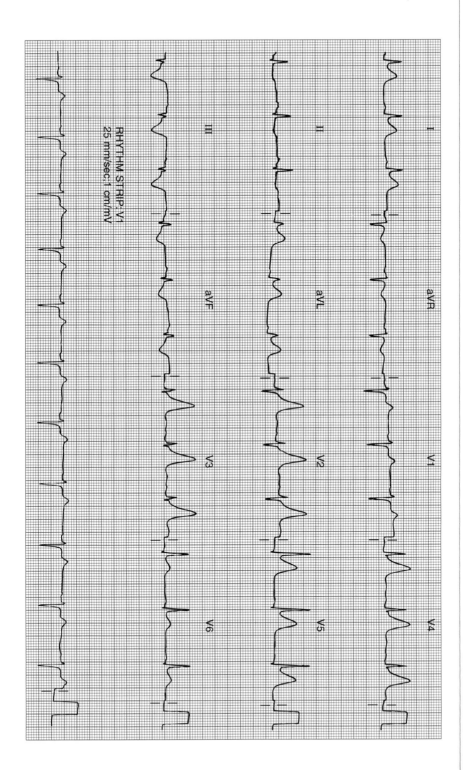

RHYTHM STRIP: V1
25 mm/sec: 1 cm/mV

ECG 4

A 46-year-old man is admitted with a depressive illness. He tells you he is on warfarin and a 'small tablet for his heart.' His ECG is shown in the figure.

What rhythm is the patient in?

What 'small tablet' do you think the patient is on?

How does this ECG affect your management of his depressive illness?

Suggested approach

The rate is about 84/min.

The rhythm is irregular.

No P waves are seen but there is some atrial activity in V1.

The rhythm is therefore coarse atrial fibrillation.

The axis is normal.

The QRS complexes are normal.

There is ST depression in V3 to V6.

There is T wave inversion in V2 to V4, and in the inferior leads (II, II, aVF).

The tablet is likely to be digoxin. The rate is atrial fibrillation and digoxin is commonly used to control the rate of this arrhythmia. The ST depression and T wave inversion on the ECG, commonly known as the 'reverse tick effect', is sometimes seen with digoxin therapy.

Since the rate is satisfactory, no other rate-controlling medication is required.

In terms of antidepressant therapy, SSRI can interact with warfarin and so I will monitor his INR and liaise with the haematologists. Tricyclic antidepressants can provoke arrhythmias, and so I will try to avoid them.

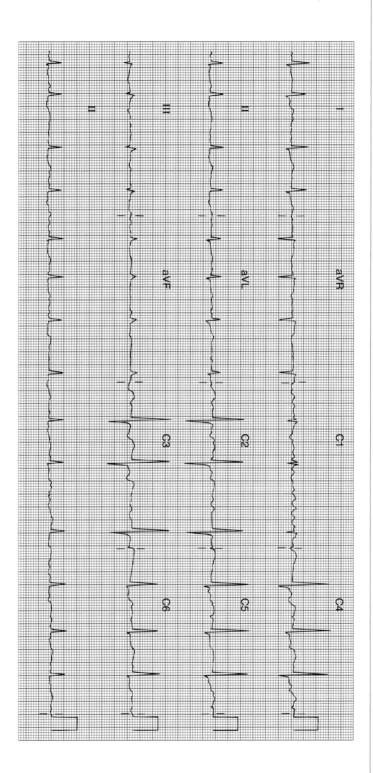

ECG 5

A 64-year-old man is admitted with a relapse of depression. He has no chest pain and his observations are satisfactory. A routine ECG is performed.

Describe the ECG.

What action do you take?

How will this ECG affect your choice of antidepressant?

Suggested approach

The rate is about 100/min and the rhythm is sinus.

P wave morphology is normal.

PR interval is 0.12 (three small squares), which is normal.

The axis is normal.

There are small Q waves in leads III and aVF.

There are pathological Q waves in V2 and V3, and the R wave in V4 is very small. There is ST elevation in V2 and V3 but there is no reciprocal ST depression in the other leads.

There is T wave inversion in the lateral leads (V5, V6, I, aVL).

The presence of pathological Q waves suggests that a full-thickness infarct occurred over 24 hours ago.

I will take a full history and do a physical examination. Since the patient is well, it is unlikely that this event is recent. However, I will repeat the ECG within 15–30 minutes just to be sure. ST elevation which persists usually indicates the presence of a left ventricular aneurysm. Since the ECG is highly abnormal, I will contact the medical registrar.

I will avoid tricyclic antidepressants in view of the risk of arrhythmia.

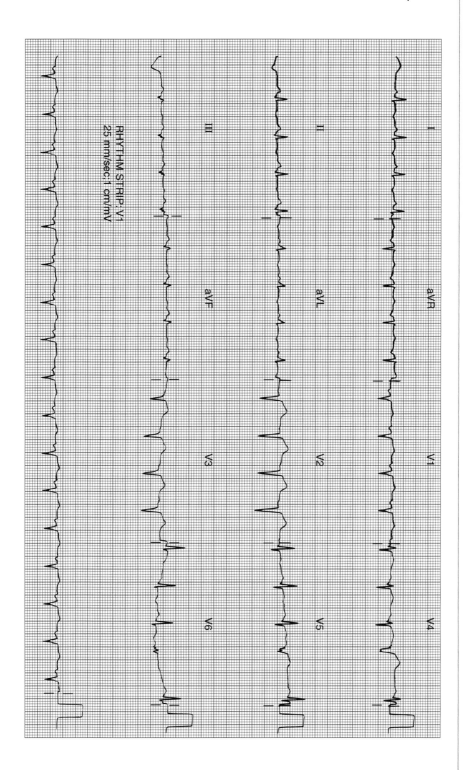

RHYTHM STRIP: V1
25 mm/sec; 1 cm/mV

ECG 6

A 45-year-old woman with a paranoid psychosis is being treated with an atypical antipsychotic drug. A routine ECG is performed.

Comment on the ECG.

Describe your initial management plan.

Suggested approach

The ECG shows a sinus bradycardia of about 55/min.

The axis is normal.

The P waves are normal.

The PR interval is about 0.14 s (3.5 small squares).

The QRS complexes and T waves are normal.

However, the QT interval is prolonged at about 560 ms (14 small squares). The QTc is 533 ms (normal is less than 420 ms). QTc is calculated by dividing the QT interval by √(R–R interval).

The long QTc is likely to be due to the atypical antipsychotic drug. This needs to be substituted with another antipsychotic drug that will not have QTc-prolonging effect. I will keep monitoring her ECG.

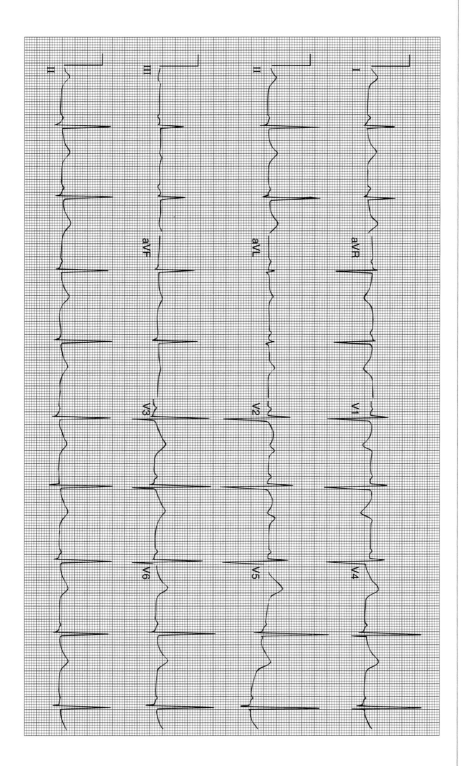

34 Elicit hallucinations

A. Michael

CONSTRUCT

The candidate demonstrates the ability to establish a rapport with a patient and to elicit hallucinations.

INSTRUCTION TO CANDIDATE

The GP has referred a middle-aged person to you with a history of hearing voices. Elicit hallucinations.

CHECKLIST

- Elementary
- Second person
- Third person
- Running commentary
- Command
- Thoughts being heard aloud
- Pseudo-hallucinations
- Visual, Lilliputian
- Olfactory, gustatory
- Tactile, somatic, vestibular
- Functional, reflex, extracampine, autoscopy
- Control over the hallucinations
- Explanation
- Effects, coping.

SUGGESTED APPROACH

Introduce the topic tactfully. Move from open-ended to closed questions.

C : *Your doctor has asked me to see you because he is concerned about you. I would like to ask you some questions. Some of them may appear a bit strange. These are questions which we ask everybody who comes to the hospital. Is that all right with you?*

I gather that you had been through a lot of stress and strain recently. When under stress sometimes people have certain unusual experiences. Have you had any such experiences?

By unusual experience, I mean, for example, hearing noises or voices when there is no one around.

Do you sometimes hear whirring sounds or see flashes of light that others can't?

Can you hear voices which others cannot hear?

Do people talk behind your back?

If the patient admits to hearing voices, ask him to describe them, how many people are there, who they are, what they say etc.

Types of auditory hallucinations

Clarify the types of auditory hallucinations.

C : *Do they speak directly to you?*

    What do they say?

    Do they speak among themselves?

    What do they talk about?

    Do these voices describe or comment upon what you are doing or thinking?

    Do the voices give you orders?

    What do they ask you to do?

    Do you feel compelled to obey them?

    Can you hear what you are thinking?

    Do the voices repeat your thoughts?

    Do they anticipate your thoughts?

Pseudo-hallucinations

Confirm if they are true or pseudo-hallucinations.

C : *Where do they come from?*

    Where do you hear them?

    Do you hear them in your mind or in your ears?

    Do you hear them as clearly as you hear me?

    Can you start or stop them?

    Do you feel that they are real or do you feel that they are just voices?

Visual Lillipution

    Are there times when you can see things that others cannot see?

    Sometimes people see small insects or tiny people. Has it ever happened to you?

    Can you elaborate on them, please?

    When do you see these things?

Gustatory, olfactory

    Have you noticed your food tasting different?

    Do you sometimes get strange or unusual smells or tastes?

    Can you tell me more about that please?

Tactile somatic, vestibular

    Some people have sensations on the body, for example insects crawling or electricity passing. Have you had any such experiences?

    What about feeling of wind blowing or electricity passing?

    Do you sometimes get the feeling that your muscles are stretched or squeezed?

    Do you sometimes feel that you are floating in the air or sinking through your bed?

    Are there any particular situations when you had these experiences?

Functional, reflex, extracampine, autoscopy

Now I want to ask you about certain things that are a bit more complicated. Don't worry if you can't understand my questions. You would understand them if you had such experiences.

Sometimes, people hear a normal sound such as someone sneezing or a car sounding its horn. When they hear such a sound, they also hear voices as if someone is talking to them. Have such things even happened to you? [Functional]

Some people report that when they have one normal sensation, they also get a different sensation. For example, when a person hears someone sneezing or a car sounding its horn, they also get pain in the head. Does this ring any bells? [Reflex]

Can you at times hear someone talking to you from miles away?

Can you ever see things happening behind your back? [Extracampine]

Have you ever seen your double?

Has it ever happened to you that you see yourself or your body walking around and doing things while you are observing what is going on? [Autoscopy]

Explanation, effects, coping

How long have you had these experiences?

What started them off?

How often do they happen lately?

Would anything make it more likely or less likely to happen?

How would you explain them?

Could it be your imagination?

How do they affect you?

How do they make you feel?

How would you cope with them?

What have you done about them?

What do you intend to do about them?

Is there anything I have missed?

Is there anything you would like to ask me?

P : Do you think I am lying?

C : *I believe you are telling the truth. You experience these things, but not others.*

P : What do you think is the problem?

C : *What you have described to me is called a xx hallucination. I will need some more information before I can tell you what it means.*

Assess premorbid personality

35

C. O'Loughlin

CONSTRUCT
The candidate demonstrates the ability to assess premorbid personality.

INSTRUCTIONS TO CANDIDATE
A 40-year-old man has made a complete recovery from an episode of severe depression. Your consultant has asked you to assess his premorbid personality.

CHECKLIST
- Introduction: explain personality, confirm the period in question
- Development, maturity, stability, employment, relationships
- Leisure, drugs, alcohol
- Ambition, fantasy life, spiritual life
- Self-confidence, self-reliance, assertiveness
- Sociability
- Mood, worries and coping
- Perfectionism, attitudes, beliefs, standards, flexibility
- Trustfulness, hostility
- Antisocial, impulsiveness
- Warmth, histrionic, borderline, attention seeking
- Summarise
- Change.

SUGGESTED APPROACH

Introduction
Explain in plain language the purpose of the interview and the concept of personality. Confirm the onset of the illness. Explain that the period in question is that before the onset of the illness.

C : *Could you tell me what kind of a person you were before you became ill?*

If I had asked your friends what sort of person you were before you became ill, what do you think they would have said?

If we had met before all this happened, how would you have come across to me then?

How would you have described yourself compared to others?

Development, maturity, stability

C : *Can you tell me about what sort of a child you were?*

How did you get on at school?

How old were you when you left home?

How easy or difficult was leaving home?

Enquire about current/last relationship, longest relationship, current and longest job. Enquire about leisure activities, hobbies and alcohol and drug use.

Ambition, fantasy life, spiritual life

C : *Before you became ill, what did you want to achieve in life?*

Did you consider yourself an ambitious person?

Did you have an active imagination?

Tell me about your daydreams in those days.

What sort of dreams did you use to have?

Did you use to have nightmares?

Did you have any religious beliefs?

Did you practise your religion? / Did you go to church etc.?

Did you find your beliefs helped you in difficult times? How?

Self-confidence, self-reliance, assertiveness

C : *How confident did you use to feel in yourself?*

How much did you usually depend on others?

When you had problems, did you sort them out yourself or did you seek help?

How comfortable did you usually feel about making a stand?

Did others often tend to dominate you?

How did you cope when the most stressful things in your life happened?

Sociability

C : *How did you usually get on with people?*

Did you use to have many friends?

How easily did you use to make friends?

Did you usually initiate a conversation?

Do you enjoy doing things in groups or alone?

Were you usually the heart and soul of the party?

How did you usually get on with your workmates?

How did you usually get on with the authorities?

Mood

C : *How did you usually feel in yourself?*

Did you usually feel cheerful or gloomy?

How often did your mood change?

Did your mood change spontaneously or in relation to events?

Did you usually hope for the best or expect the worst?

Do your family and friends generally consider you as a moody person?

Worries and coping, avoidance, dependence

C : *Before becoming ill, how did you generally cope with life?*

Did you use to worry a lot?

With whom did you share your worries?

Did you use to find life too stressful to cope with?

How did you usually feel when things did not happen the way you expected?

How often did you worry about people not liking you?

Did you find making decisions difficult?

Did you like taking responsibilities?

Did you like to be the leader or the follower?

Perfectionism, attitudes, beliefs, standards, flexibility

C : *Would you have described yourself as an organised person?*

Enquire about standards at home and at work, being fussy, house-proud, neat and tidy.

C : *Did you use to have any strong views about moral standards?*

Did people generally consider you as someone who adjusted to change?

Did others influence you easily?

Antisocial, impulsiveness

C : *How was your temper before you became ill?*

Have you been in trouble with the police?

Have you ever been violent?

Did others consider you as irresponsible?

Were these behaviours present most of the time or only certain times, for example when you were stressed or after you had had a few drinks?

How quickly did you use to make decisions?

Trustfulness, hostility

C : *How did you find people in general?*

Did you generally trust people?

How did you use to take criticism?

If you found something wrong, would you criticise it immediately?

Would you have been concerned about offending others before you make a comment?

Warmth, histrionic, borderline, attention seeking

C : *Before you became ill, did you usually display your feelings or keep them to yourself?*

Did you have many close relationships?

Did you often crave attention?

Did people feel that you were a bit overemotional?

Were you afraid of being abandoned?

How did you use to respond when in crisis?

Have you ever harmed yourself? (Taken an overdose, cut yourself ...)

Summary and change

Summarise the salient features and ask for his comments.

Enquire how his usual nature has changed since the onset of the illness.

36 Explain psychogeriatric services

F. Lazaro-Perlado

CONSTRUCT

The candidate demonstrates the ability to establish a rapport with a distressed relative and to explain the current practice in psychogeriatrics, stressing close working relationships with the family and a multidisciplinary approach.

INSTRUCTIONS TO CANDIDATE

The daughter of an elderly man recently admitted informally to your unit, suffering from a dementing illness of moderate severity, does not see any reason for the admission and would like her father discharged to his home immediately. She seems to be upset and is demanding to speak to the doctor in charge. Explain the situation and management plan.

CHECKLIST

- Introduction and reassurance
- Circumstances leading to admission
- Aims of the admission
- Multidisciplinary assessment
- Home assessment
- Working with the family and the patient
- Discharge planning
- Role of the community psychiatric nurse
- Conclusion.

SUGGESTED APPROACH

It would be helpful to meet the relative together with a senior nurse. Introduce yourself and your colleague.

C : *Thanks very much for asking to see us. I can understand that the present situation can be overwhelming, but let me tell you that we have your father's well-being in mind and I can promise you that we'd like to discharge him as soon as possible ...*

Circumstances leading to admission

C : *I am not sure if you were aware of why your father agreed to be admitted. To avoid any confusion, let me explain what happened ... Although we tried to support your father at home, the situation deteriorated and as he was putting himself at risk we suggested admission to hospital as the next step ...*

Aims of the admission

C : *... so that we could review the situation and find out the reasons for his deterioration. Sometimes something trivial such as an infection in his waterworks or consti-*

pation can cause such deterioration. We will also need to assess his dementia in depth, as the present situation could be the natural course of his illness. We need to assess his current needs and also plan for the future, in order to discharge him with the support and care he will need, and make arrangements for regular reviews in the future, so that his care matches his changing needs.

Multidisciplinary assessment

C : I would like to take the opportunity to briefly outline how we work as a team and what role different professionals have. As doctors, we'll monitor your father's mental state to make sure that he is not feeling, for example, particularly sad or unduly concerned about issues that wouldn't normally bother him, or become easily irritable. We'll be able to assess more deeply the extent of his cognitive deficits and its causes. Where appropriate we'll prescribe medication and monitor its side effects. We also look after his physical health and have ready access to services of other specialties.

The nursing staff will help us to monitor his mental state and physical health, but they would also get to know him better, and his preferences. They'll be able to monitor his level of functioning in everyday life activities, his mobility, offer support and they'll be more than happy to update you on his progress and help you with any of your concerns.

The occupational therapists assess in detail what his needs would be in what we call the activities of daily living, such as dressing, bathing, feeding, toileting, washing, cooking and travelling capabilities, and detect problems in other areas such as mobility and interaction with others. They also run a variety of activities on the ward which we encourage patients to attend, and can also offer advice in different techniques such as anxiety management.

The physiotherapists will assess and up to a degree treat problems related to his joints and movements. They advise about ambulatory aids such as sticks or Zimmer frames.

The psychologists in our team advise about psychological treatments and also carry out tests for memory and related problems. In essence, they would be able to tell us in more detail what cognitive problems your father has and to what extent.

In due course you'll meet with one of our social workers. They provide help and advice in different matters, ranging from help to set up a direct debit to pay the gas bill for example, to being responsible to set up the care package. Where appropriate they advise the relatives and patient about residential placements, also looking into the financial aspect of it.

As you can see, our assessment is a complex and thorough process in which different professionals are involved.

Home assessment

C : Sometimes people perform differently when in an unfamiliar environment, so we like to assess how the patient does when at home. To this effect we organise what we call a home assessment. Usually the occupational therapists do it, but other professionals, like the social workers, sometimes attend. During these assessments we collect valuable information about how the patient behaves in a familiar environment and what needs he has. We also advise about complementary apparatus for specific purposes, such as a stair-lift or modification to the bathroom for people with mobility problems.

Working with the family and the patient

C : *I would like to stress that all along this process we constantly seek the opinion of our patients and their families. I like to describe our work as a dynamic process in which feedback from the patients and relatives is actively sought.*

Discharge planning

C : *Once our assessment has been completed we'll meet and share our thoughts with you. We would have identified all your father's needs and we will explain how these needs can be fulfilled, by setting up what we call a care plan. We would advise as to where the patient will gain the best quality of life. In some cases this would mean no change in accommodation, but in others supervised accommodation (warden controlled) or residential placement. In any case we will design an individually tailored plan that will cover all the needs. It can include things like morning calls to help getting up, washing, dressing and supervising medication, meals on wheels, evening calls, sitting-in carers, attendance at activities in the community or even planned respite admissions. It goes without saying that your views will be taken into account.*

In the care plan we'll also include regular reviews in the future, and where appropriate follow-up by one of our community psychiatric nurses.

Role of the community psychiatric nurse

C : *Sometimes patients need to be monitored in the community with regard to mood, behavioural difficulties, gradual deterioration of dementia, side effects of medication, administration of long-acting drugs etc. So while in hospital we introduce them to the community psychiatric nurse (CPN) who will carry this out. Another advantage is that this creates a fast link to medical staff or other professionals in case this is needed. The CPN can also provide support and put you in contact with associations, such as the Alzheimer's Society, which can be of great help.*

Conclusion

C : *Well, I hope that our conversation has been of help and you can now see the way we work and what we do. As you know, I'm the ward doctor and I'll be happy to see you again if need be. I am going to pass on your concerns to the consultant responsible for your father's care and tell him about our conversation. I'm sure that he'll be happy to talk to you but you'll need to make an appointment. You can get the contact number from the nursing staff. Please do not hesitate to contact me if I can be of any help, and also be aware that the nurses will be happy to discuss any of your concerns.*

Explain risks of excess alcohol intake

M. London

CONSTRUCT

The candidate demonstrates the ability to establish a rapport with and to explain the risks of excess alcohol intake to a person who drinks excessively. The candidate uses this session to motivate the person to look at his drinking pattern and to consider the options.

INSTRUCTIONS TO CANDIDATE

His general practitioner refers Mr Tennant, a 40-year-old builder, to you because his wife is concerned about his alcohol intake. He has been drinking about 60 pints of lager a week for the past few years. Recently, he has had episodes when he had no memory of his behaviour the previous night, even though he was behaving rather normally. He denied withdrawal symptoms or any other adverse effects. His liver function tests have been normal. Explain the presenting problem and the other risks of excess alcohol intake.

CHECKLIST

- Introduction
- Presenting problem
- Neurological and other physical aspects
- Psychiatric
- Family, social, occupational, legal
- Enquire if he recognises/has experienced any of the complications
- Summary
- Suggest involving family
- Avoid lecturing the patient.

SUGGESTED APPROACH

C : *Hello Mr Tennant, what brings you here today?*

P : My doctor and my wife think that I am losing my marbles. I usually drink about 60 pints a week. It has been going up slowly over the past few years, but I drink only ordinary-strength lager and I never get drunk or get into trouble. The problem is that some mornings I can't remember what I was doing the previous night.

C : *Sixty pints would be about 120 units a week, more than four times the safe limit. All right. Can you tell me more about your memory problem?*

P : This problem started only recently. Some mornings when I get up I can't remember where I was or what I have been doing the previous night. I have gone back to the pub and asked the landlady if there was any problem the previous night. She would say that everything was fine and that I have always been a gentleman. It puzzles me.

C : *I think you are describing 'alcoholic blackouts'.*

P : But doctor, I don't get drunk or fall over. I have never been unconscious.

C : *You are correct. In blackouts, one drinks the usual amount, behaves perfectly well, finds his way home and goes to sleep. When he wakes up the next morning he can't remember anything that happened the previous night. Alcoholic blackouts are often the first signs of alcohol seriously affecting the brain.*

With your level of drinking, it is hardly surprising. I think it will be useful for us to talk about things that often happen to people who drink excessively.

Tell me how alcohol affects the brain.

P : I think some people go senile with too much alcohol.

C : *You are correct. Alcohol is toxic to the brain cells. When people drink too much for too long, the nerve cells take the toll. They die off. This can cause memory loss and dementia. In one particular type of memory problem called Korsakoff's, people can't learn anything new. They forget everything they have seen, heard or done within a few seconds.*

Alcohol also affects the nerves outside the brain, for example in the legs and arms. This affects the sensation. We call this peripheral neuropathy.

Tell me about what alcohol can do to other parts of the body.

P : Well, in people with a weak liver, it can affect the liver.

C : *You are right. The liver has to work hard to get the alcohol out of the body. Even the healthiest liver has a limit. After some time the liver becomes exhausted and it starts failing. This can cause hepatitis and jaundice. It then starts shrinking, causing cirrhosis of the liver, and kills the person.*

What else can alcohol do to your body?

P : Alcohol can cause a burning stomach.

C : *Yes. Alcohol irritates the stomach walls and can cause gastritis. It can make stomach ulcers worse. In fact, alcohol affects every system in the body. Alcohol can damage the food pipe and cause massive bleeding. It can damage the pancreas and interfere with blood glucose. Alcohol can cause heart problems. Alcohol is the commonest cause for people ending up in casualty with broken bones or head injury. Alcohol is a very common cause of premature death.*

Do you think alcohol can cause any mental health problems?

P : Yes, hangover.

C : *Not only that. Excess drinking itself is a mental health problem. People often get tolerant to and hooked on alcohol.*

Have you had difficulty cutting down because you get little effect or just because you like the taste?

Do you get shakes when you try to cut down?

Have you heard voices or seen things when you missed your drinks?

How often do you crave alcohol?

These suggest alcohol withdrawal. This can progress to something called delirium tremens. This is a medical emergency.

Some people hear frightening voices all the time.

What do you think alcohol does to people's mood?

P : Alcohol makes people relaxed and confident. That's why they drink.

C : *You are correct. Alcohol relaxes, but only within a certain limit. Beyond that, it causes problems. Alcohol is a very common cause of depression, anxiety and sleep problems. Many people who take overdoses and kill themselves have an alcohol problem and they do so while drunk*

What does alcohol do to people's sex lives?

P : Well, alcohol gives them confidence.

C : *In fact, alcohol causes all sorts of sexual problems, including loss of erection and sexual jealousy.*

How does alcohol affect family life?

P : Well, my wife is very worried. She often nags me. Sometimes we row.

C : *I think she is right to worry about you. Alcohol is a very common reason for domestic violence and family break-ups.*

Have you had any problems at work because of your drinking?

P : Yes, I miss work some Mondays and I had a final warning.

C : *How much of your earnings would you spend on drinks?*

P : My wife nags me about money too.

C : *Often alcohol becomes the most expensive thing in people's lives. Many people get into serious debt because of their drinking.*

What other harm do you think alcohol can cause?

P : We have talked about too many things. I can't think of anything else.

C : *Well, there are many people with only one conviction in their lives, and that would be for drunk driving or drunk and disorderly behaviour.*

Now, tell me some good things about alcohol.

P : Well, for me the pub has been my life for a very long time.

C : *I agree, but probably there are many other things in life you have been missing out on all these years. It may be a good idea to look at them also.*

Is there anything else you would like to talk about?

P : No doctor, I've had enough.

C : *Let me sum up what we have discussed. You have been drinking far too much alcohol for a long time. It has started affecting your brain. If you continue, you are likely to get problems with every system in your body including your brain, liver, stomach, pancreas, heart etc. You are likely to become dependent on alcohol. You may get withdrawal shakes and delirium if you stop drinking suddenly. You are likely to get depression, anxiety, sleep problems and sexual problems. Alcohol can cause family break-ups, work and money problems and problems with the law. It is time to do something about it. It is not easy, but we can help you.*

Do you have any questions?

P : No. Thank you.

C : *I will give you some reading materials. I would like you to go home, think about it and discuss it with your wife. I will make an appointment to see you and your wife together to discuss plans. Is that all right with you?*

38 Elicit negative cognitions in depression

F. Iqbal

CONSTRUCT

The candidate demonstrates the ability to establish a rapport with a depressed patient and elicit negative cognitions.

INSTRUCTIONS TO CANDIDATE

Elicit negative cognitions in a 42-year-old man suffering from depression. He is married with two children and works as an accounts assistant in an accounting firm. He was referred by the GP for an assessment.

CHECKLIST

- Introduction
- Negative view of self
- Negative view of world
- Negative view of future
- Consider nihilistic delusions
- Consider suicide risk
- Summarise.

SUGGESTED APPROACH

C : *I am Dr ____ , and I am a psychiatrist. I understand that you saw your GP as you have been feeling a bit depressed lately and it was his suggestion that you see me.*

P : Well, I didn't really want to waste your time but my doctor thought that it was important.

C : *I wondered if you would be able to tell me how things have been for you.*

P : You see, doctor, the thing is that everything is just a big mess right now. It's just that I feel absolutely awful. I can't sleep, I can't work and I'm always in a terrible mood – shouting at the kids – It's just terrible. [Negative view of world/present]

C : *Sounds like you're having a rough time, but tell me how you feel about yourself.*

P : To be frank, pretty awful. I am just not able to manage anything. No matter what I do, no matter how hard I try, I always seem to mess things up. I've been a failure all of my life and that's how it will always be. [Negative view of self]

C : *It sounds like you are quite convinced that you are a failure, but I am not quite sure why you consider yourself to be a failure.*

P : I screw up everything I do. I lie in bed most of the time doing nothing and the times that I come out I shout at the kids when it's not their fault anyway. I'm a terrible husband. My wife, she's a good woman. She deserves better. [Negative view of self]

C : *Is that something that they've told you?*

P : No, they tell me that they love me, but how can anyone love somebody like me? [Worthlessness]

C : *You've mentioned how you feel about things at home but I wondered how things were outside home – at work and with friends?*

P : At work, well, to tell you the truth I think I'm going to lose my job and I don't blame my boss for it. I've been off work for some time but even before that I wasn't coping and I was just causing problems. You see, it's quite a responsible position and the truth is that I was never really up to the job in the first place.

Friends – well, I don't see them anymore. There's not much point. Who would want to spend time with a miserable person like me? So I stopped going out with them. [Negative view of self and world]

C : *How were other people getting on with you at work?*

P : Well, generally they were polite. But you know how things are. People talk about you when you aren't around. It's just how things are these days. I am sure that most people from the office will be pleased to see my back. I'm not a very sociable person so I suppose they are right. [Negative view of self and world]

C : *From your account it seems that you're having a difficult time and I wonder whether you blame yourself for these difficulties.*

P : I don't think there is any one else to blame. I suppose I could try harder, being a bit more caring towards my family and friends and pushing myself a bit more at work, but I haven't and I can't. I'm just a very weak person. [Negative view of self]

C : *It seems to me that you blame yourself for a lot of things and I wondered whether you blame yourself for the depression?*

P : There are things that I've done, and I shouldn't have. If I were a bit stronger, I wouldn't be depressed, would I? I think that I've just given up and I am not trying anymore, and that is not fair on others. [Self-blame]

C : *I understand that you have been feeling a bit low for the past couple of months and I wondered whether you felt the same about yourself, your family, work, friends, before that, when you weren't feeling low?*

P : Not at the time, but I suppose that I've been living a lie for a long time. It's just that now I realise that I've always been like this. [Negative view of self and past]

C : *You've told me that at the moment things feel quite bad but I wondered how you feel about the future?*

P : I can't think that far ahead.

C : *Do you feel that things might change and get better?*

P : I suppose there is a chance but, doctor, at the moment it seems that things can only get worse. I can't really see things getting better. [Negative view of future/hopelessness]

C : *Do you think that you can be helped in anyway?*

P : No, doctor. [Helplessness]

C : *Do you feel that people around you might be able to help you through this difficult time?*

P : Maybe, who knows? I don't think they can, I think things are beyond that now. [Helplessness]

Assess risk of suicide (see 'Assess suicide risk').

Summarise

C : *Now you've told me that things have been pretty awful for you and you feel pretty dreadful about yourself, feeling a bit like a failure and blaming yourself, for the illness, for letting your friends, family and work colleagues down, and also that you can't see things getting any better.*

But I was also thinking that you came here to see me and you've been able to talk about how you feel, and I wondered whether you felt that we might be able to help you and get things sorted.

P : It's been a bit of a relief being able to talk about things to somebody who can understand. [Checking for helplessness in the context]

C : *It might take some time but hopefully we can figure out the best way of getting things back on track.*

P : Sounds reasonable.

C : *I shall arrange to see you again and we shall be able to discuss things in detail.*

Do you have any questions?

Is there anything else that you'd like to tell me?

P : No, doctor, but thanks for listening. I really do appreciate your help.

Assess suicide risk

39

N. Omara

CONSTRUCT
The candidate demonstrates the ability to establish a rapport with a young woman who recently took an overdose and to assess the current risk of suicide.

INSTRUCTIONS TO CANDIDATE
Assess the current risk of suicide in a 20-year-old woman admitted to the medical ward following an overdose.

CHECKLIST
- Empathy and understanding
- Recent attempt: Precipitating factors, planning, final acts, precautions, danger-ousness, expectation of fatality, help seeking, how found, attitude to the act, previous attempts
- Current risk: Current problems, mood, hopelessness, suicidal thoughts and plans, preparation, lethality of the proposed method, reasons for not proceed-ing, intent, coping patterns, help and support, alcohol and drug use
- Action plan
- Summary.

NB: In clinical practise, liaise with the referring doctors and the ward staff.

SUGGESTED APPROACH

Introduction
C : *I gather that you had been through a tough time. Can you tell me what happened?*
I know it is very distressing, but can you tell me about the overdose, please?

RECENT ATTEMPT

Precipitating factors
C : *What made you think of harming yourself?*
What sorts of things have been worrying you?
Have you suffered any setbacks lately?
Do you have any relationship problems?
Do you have any problems at work?
Do you have financial worries or health problems?
What was the last straw?

Planning

C : *How long did you think about it before you actually took the overdose?*

Do you know of anyone else who did something like this recently?

Final acts

C : *What preparations did you make?*

Did you leave a note?

Did you bid farewell to anybody?

Precautions

C : *What did you do to prevent someone spoiling your plans?*

Dangerousness

C : *What tablets did you take?*

How did you get them?

What did you think might happen?

Did you take all the tablets or did you leave a few behind?

Did you take anything else with the tablets, for example alcohol?

Help seeking

C : *What did you do after taking the overdose?*

How were you found?

How did you feel when you were found?

Previous attempts

C : *How many times has something like this happened in the past?*

Can you tell me about the worst one?

CURRENT RISK

Current problems

C : *Did your problems change in any way after the overdose?*

Have any new problems started since?

What else is bothering you?

Mood and hopelessness

C : *How do you feel in yourself?*

How bad is it?

How do you see the future?

Do you still feel that life is not worth living?

Suicidal thoughts and plans

C : *Do you wish you were dead?*

Do you have thoughts of harming yourself in any way?

What do you think you might do?

Have you made any plans?

Have you mentally rehearsed a plan?

When are you intending to do it?

What prevents you from doing it?

How do you think it will affect your loved ones?

Have you thought of doing anything to help them out?

How dangerous do you think this would be?

Preparation

C : *Have you made any preparations?*

Have you told anybody about it?

Coping patterns, help and supports

C : *What do you usually do when there is a problem? How do you usually cope?*

Who do you share your worries with?

Do you get any help?

In the past, did anyone offer you any help?

How did you find it?

Enquire about contact with RELATE and the Citizens Advice Bureau (CAB).

ALCOHOL AND DRUGS

Enquire about current use.

ACTION PLAN

C : *If you are discharged today, will someone be with you at least for the next few days?*

When things go wrong, you try hard to cope. What is the first thing that you do which ends up in an overdose?

Some people, when they feel desperate, start drinking, and finally end up with an overdose. Would that be true in your case too?

Next time when you feel desperate, could you ring my colleague at the CMHT?

I would like to see you on two more occasions, about 2 weeks later and then 6 weeks later. Is that all right with you?

I would like you to contact RELATE and the CAB today.

I know you are trying hard to sort out your life. We will try our best to help you.

Is there anything you would like to ask me?

SUMMARY

C : *Let me summarise what we discussed. You have been struggling hard to cope with your problems. When you feel desperate you start drinking and this ends up with an overdose and your problems get even worse. You are very keen to do something about it. I will introduce you to my colleague at the CMHT today. When you are in crisis next time, you will contact her rather than turn to the bottle or think of an overdose. You will contact RELATE and the CAB today. I will see you again after 2 weeks and again after 6 weeks. We will try our best to help you. I will give you all the telephone numbers in writing.*

REFERENCES

General Hospital Management of Deliberate Self Harm. Royal College of Psychiatrists Council Report 32

Managing Deliberate Self-harm in Young People. Royal College of Psychiatrists Council Report 64

Explain electroconvulsive therapy

M. Stevens

CONSTRUCT

The candidate demonstrates the ability to establish a rapport with an elderly patient who has a moderately severe depression that has not responded to two different antidepressants. The candidate explains the nature, advantages and disadvantages of electroconvulsive therapy (ECT) to the patient with a view to getting informed consent.

INSTRUCTIONS TO CANDIDATE

A 67-year-old man with a major depressive disorder – severe with somatic symptoms – has not responded to paroxetine 50 mg and later amitriptyline 175 mg, both for 6 weeks each. Your consultant has asked you to discuss ECT with the patient and to get consent.

CHECKLIST

● Be considerate
● Explain the diagnosis, treatment options, prognosis and rationale for ECT
● Explore what he knows about ECT, correct misapprehensions
● Explain the procedure, who will administer it and the mechanism of action
● Explain the benefits, disadvantages, possible complications and uncertainties
● Offer written information and encourage discussing with family and friends
● Do not press for immediate consent, respect the patient's decision to refuse.

SUGGESTED APPROACH

C : *Thank you Mr ___ for agreeing to see me. I would like to discuss possible changes in your treatment with you. Is this a convenient time to do so?*

P : Yes, that's fine.

C : *Thank you. Please interrupt me if I am not clear or if you have any questions. As you know, you have been suffering from a severe depression. So far we have tried two different antidepressants. Despite experiencing unpleasant side effects, you co-operated fully with the treatment, but, unfortunately, your depression has not improved. Indeed, sometimes you appear to feel even worse. Therefore, I think it would be a good idea to consider what other treatments we might try.*

P : What other treatments are there?

C : *The main kinds of treatment for depressive illness are psychological or physical. Physical treatments include various antidepressant drugs as well as ECT.*

P : What about counselling?

C : *I presume you mean psychological treatments. They are generally more useful in milder depressions. Currently, your depression is too severe for you to benefit from* *them. We can surely consider them when your depression improves with medication or ECT. Once you have recovered, they can also help reduce the chances of depression coming back.*

P : What about another drug?

C : *With regard to medication, we could try yet another antidepressant drug, combine an antidepressant with a mood stabiliser such as lithium or try a combination of antidepressants. However, you may have to wait for up to 6 weeks to know whether the new drug is effective, and there is the possibility of new side effects. Most importantly, we are worried about your depression worsening, and want to relieve your continued suffering as soon as possible. We know that ECT usually works more quickly than medication and will often work when antidepressants have failed.*

P : So are you telling me that I must have ECT?

C : *No. We don't want to tell you what you must have. We want to discuss the options with you and to make a joint decision about how best to treat your depression.*

P : ECT is shock treatment, isn't it?

C : *Yes, in one sense. ECT stands for electroconvulsive therapy. This means that while the patient is asleep under anaesthesia, a small electric shock is given to provoke a convulsion. However, the patient never feels the shock, as they sometimes may when electric shocks are given to treat other medical conditions such as irregular heart rhythms. What have you heard about or read about ECT?*

P : I have heard that ECT is a barbaric treatment.

C : *I appreciate that some people are strongly opposed to the idea of ECT. Most of the objections are based on treatments given several years ago, with older equipment and when less was known about the best doses and when anaesthesia was less advanced. ECT has become very sophisticated over the last few years. Nowadays most patients who have had ECT are willing to have another course if necessary and some even ask for further treatment before their doctors suggest it!*

P : How does it work?

C : *As you know, various chemical messengers are involved in controlling the functions of the brain. When some of these chemicals, especially serotonin, noradrenaline and dopamine, change in certain ways, depression results. Antidepressant drugs and ECT work by normalising them.*

P : Since the medication has not worked, why should ECT work?

C : *Research has shown that ECT usually works faster than medication, especially in more severe depressions. More importantly, ECT often works even when medication has not worked. In the most severe illnesses when patients' lives are at risk, we use ECT without waiting to try medication. In patients in whom it may be risky to try or who are unable to tolerate high doses and combinations of medication, ECT is a safe and effective choice.*

P : What are the chances that I might die during the procedure?

C : *Very low. The risk of death is less than if you have a tooth removed under general anaesthesia. It is less than one in 50,000 treatments. All anaesthetics carry a slight risk but we attempt to minimise this by giving you a detailed physical examination, blood tests and a heart tracing beforehand.*

P : What side effects will I have?

C : *The side effects are usually mild and short lasting. You may have some muscle pains, nausea or headache immediately after treatment. You will have no memory of the treatment and you may feel slightly confused for an hour or two. Your memory for the period immediately before, during, and immediately after the treatment may be affected. You may have difficulties with some personal memories such as telephone numbers or names of familiar people. This usually clears up within a few weeks.*

P : My memory is not very good now. I am very worried about making it worse.

C : *We carefully calculate the lowest, efficient dose for each individual patient and give treatment only twice a week and reduce this to once a week if confusion becomes a problem. If ECT causes memory problems, instead of giving the electrical stimulus bilaterally across both temples, we can give it unilaterally to just one side of the head.*

P : What will happen if I consent to treatment?

C : *An anaesthetist will examine you to decide whether you are fit for a short anaesthetic. Prior to treatment you will have to fast overnight. On the morning of treatment we will escort you to the ECT clinic. There will be an anaesthetist, a psychiatrist and at least one nurse present. You will lie on a couch and be asked to breathe some oxygen while we attach equipment to you to monitor your blood pressure, heart tracing and brainwaves. We will then give you an injection of a short-acting anaesthetic and a muscle relaxant. Once you are fast asleep we will place two electrodes on your head and pass a small electric current. This will produce seizure-like activity in your brain lasting less than a minute. Within a few minutes, the anaesthetic will wear off and you will regain consciousness. You may feel rather muzzy headed at first. There will be a member of staff with you throughout the procedure. You will normally be able to have your lunch on your own.*

P : Who will pass the current?

C : *A psychiatrist who is trained and experienced in giving ECT. This will be the consultant responsible for the ECT clinic or a junior psychiatrist working under his supervision.*

P : How many ECTs will I have to have?

C : *There is no fixed number. Usually people with depression need about six to eight ECTs, but some patients recover after three or four treatments and, rarely, some need more than eight. We will assess you for improvement, side effects and the need for further treatment after each ECT.*

P : What if I say no?

C : *We will respect your decision. We will continue to try to get you better with drugs. If you are not getting better, we will discuss the options again.*

P : So what do you want me to do now?

C : *I will give you some written information. I would like you to go through this and discuss it with your family and friends and your nurses on the ward.*

If you wish, you may have a second opinion. I would be happy to discuss any further questions with you or, if you like, to see you with your family or friends.

If you decide to try ECT, please let me know. Then I will ask you to sign a consent form and I will make arrangements to start treatment. Please remember that, even after giving written consent, at any time you can change your mind.

41 | Assess extrapyramidal side effects

S. N. Thiyagesh

CONSTRUCT

The candidate demonstrates the ability to assess extrapyramidal symptoms in a patient on antipsychotic medication.

INSTRUCTIONS TO CANDIDATE

A community psychiatric nurse (CPN) has asked you to see a patient who is on antipsychotic medication because he is complaining of side effects. Examine the patient for extrapyramidal side effects.

CHECKLIST

- Unobtrusive observation
- Introduction and history
- Do a focused examination
- Explain physical examination and each task
- Look for hypokinesia, rigidity, abnormal movements and akathisia.

SUGGESTED APPROACH

Observe the patient in the waiting room, walking into the consultation room, sitting down and talking.

Observe for:

- Decreased expressive movements/mask-like appearance of face
- Simian/stooped posture
- Slurring or poverty of speech
- Pooling and drooling of saliva.

Look for abnormal movements:

- Tremor: repetitive, rhythmic and regular. Best seen by placing a paper on the hand
- Choreic movements: rapid, objectively purposeless, irregular and spontaneous
- Athetoid movements: slow, irregular and serpentine.

Consider a chaperone.

Introduction

C : *Your CPN has asked me to see you because you are experiencing some side effects from the medication. Am I right?*

Could you tell me what medication you are taking now?

When was the last time the type or the dose of medication was changed?

Now, could you tell me about the problems you have been having with the medication?

Have you noticed any unusual or uncomfortable movements anywhere on your body?

Has anyone else noticed any unusual movements in your face, hands or feet?

Do your eyes ever roll up or your face or tongue go into a painful spasm?

Are you experiencing any restlessness in your legs?

Enquire how severe they are and how much they interfere with his activities.

C : *I would like to examine you. Is that alright with you?*

Ask the patient to sit on the chair with hands on his knees, legs slightly apart and feet on the floor. Then ask him to hang his hands down unsupported. Look for abnormal movements.

Ask the patient to open his mouth. Look for any twitching movements (writhing) of the tongue in the resting position and when asked to protrude the tongue.

Demonstrate to the patient tapping the thumb with each finger as rapidly as possible. Ask the patient to do the same. Normally one would be able to tap 40–50 times in 15 seconds.

Look for inability to remain sitting down or the need to get up and pace up and down.

Ask the patient to stand up. Look for truncal unsteadiness and abnormal movements.

Ask the patient to walk a few steps, turn and return to his chair. Do this twice.

Look for reduced swinging of arms, slow walking, short steps, festination, shuffling etc.

Ask the patient to extend both his arms out in front with palms facing down and fingers spread out as far as possible. Look for abnormal movements.

C : *Can you raise your arms, like me, to shoulder height and then let them fall by your side?*

Look for any slowness, as the arms should normally hit the sides with a gentle slap.

Take the patient's arm in one hand and clasp his elbow with your other hand. Move the patient's upper arm to and fro and check for degree of resistance. Repeat with the other arm.

Flex and extend the patient's elbow joint and check the rigidity.

Flex and extend the patient's wrists and check for rigidity. Check rigidity also on ulnar and radial deviation.

Distract the patient by asking him to copy on the other arm what you are doing on this arm. Examine the joints in a random fashion in order to avoid the subject concentrating on a particular joint. Do remember to examine both arms.

Ask the patient to sit on an examination table with his legs able to swing freely. Grasp the ankle and raise it until the knee is partially extended. Allow it to fall. Observe for resistance to falling and diminished swinging.

Thank the patient and explain that you have completed the examination. Enquire if the patient has any queries or worries

Explain, briefly, positive and negative findings.

Explain your management plan, its rationale and the likely benefits. Thank the patient again and ask if he has any further queries

FURTHER READING

Guy W 1976 Abnormal Involuntary Movement Scale. In ECDEU Assessment Manual for Psychopharmacology (rev edn). US Department of Health, Education and Welfare, Washington, DC, pp 534-537

Munetz MR, Benjamin S 1988 How to examine patients using the Abnormal Involuntary Movement Scale. Hosp Commun Psychiatry 39: 1172–1177

Simpson GM, Angus JW 1970 A rating scale for extrapyramidal side effects. Acta Psychiat Scand, 212: 11–19

Request an EEG

42

S. Bhandari

CONSTRUCT

The candidate demonstrates the ability to discuss the risk of seizures and their prevention and management with a colleague.

INSTRUCTIONS TO CANDIDATE

Your patient is on clozapine 600 mg daily. You want to increase it further. Ring the EEG department and explain why you need an EEG for this patient.

The EEG consultant is keen to discuss the EEG changes with clozapine.

CHECKLIST

- Seizure risk dose dependent
- Risk is 4–5% >600 mg
- Risk factors: history of seizures, head injury and organic brain damage
- Risk increases with faster titration of dosage
- EEG changes dependent on plasma levels.

SUGGESTED APPROACH

C : *Hello, I am Dr ____ , an SHO in Psychiatry. I would like to refer a patient for an EEG.*

N : Could you tell me the indication for an EEG, please?

C : *This patient has schizophrenia. He is on clozapine 600 mg. We are planning to increase his dose of clozapine to above 600 mg.*

N : Do all patients on clozapine need an EEG?

C : *Not all patients on clozapine require an EEG. It is only when we increase the dose above 600 mg that we get an EEG.*

N : Can you explain the rationale please?

C : *The main reason is that clozapine increases the risk of seizures and this risk is dose dependent. At lower doses the risk is about 2%. At dosages of 600 mg/day and above the risk is between 4% and 5%.*

N : Are there any specific risk factors for seizures in patients on clozapine?

C : *Age, sex or duration of treatment does not affect the risk. A history of seizures and history of head injury or other organic brain damage does increase the risk.*

N : Does this patient have any of the above risk factors?

C : *No, he does not.*

N : Is there anything you can do to reduce the risk of seizures?

C : *Yes, we need to titrate the dose of clozapine upwards slowly as we have done in this case. Even at lower doses, fast titration upwards tends to increase the risk of seizures.*

We can also monitor clozapine levels. This is because the risk increases at plasma levels above 350 ng/ml.

N : What are the kinds of EEG changes you are looking for?

C : *EEG changes occur in 75% and paroxysmal discharges in 40% of patients on clozapine. The changes include diffuse slowing and sharp waves. I would like to rule out evidence for any paroxysmal activity.*

N : What are the types of seizures most likely to occur?

C : *Tonic–clonic seizures are the commonest type although myoclonic seizures have also been reported.*

N : Are all patients who show the changes likely to get seizures?

C : *Actually EEG changes after clozapine are quite common but seizures are rare. Therefore we hope to identify those patients most likely to develop seizures.*

N : Do you discontinue the medication if we find EEG abnormalities?

C : *Not usually. We have two options. We can either reduce the dose or add anti-convulsants.*

N : What anticonvulsant would you use?

C : *We prefer using sodium valproate. We avoid carbamazepine because it increases the risk of haematological side effects.*

N : I gather that many other antipsychotic drugs also cause seizures.

C : *Yes, you are correct. Haloperidol, zuclopenthixol, quetiapine, amisulpride and sulpiride have only minimal epileptogenic potential. Thioridazine, chlorpromazine and loxapine can cause convulsions at therapeutic doses.*

N : Tell me about the other new drugs, please.

C : *Yes, I am coming to that. Zotepine has a dose-related seizures risk, especially above 300 mg/day. There is little information about risperidone and olanzapine.*

N : That was very helpful. We would be glad to arrange an EEG quickly. I appreciate that you discussed the case with me rather than just sending me a written referral.

C : *Thank you.*

Elicit depersonalisation

R. Raguram

CONSTRUCT

The candidate demonstrates the ability to establish a rapport with a patient and elicit depersonalisation symptoms.

INSTRUCTIONS TO CANDIDATE

The GP has referred a young man to you with persistent complaints of a feeling of being unreal. Elicit depersonalisation.

CHECKLIST

- Make the patient comfortable
- Depersonalisation
- Derealisation
- Accompanying symptoms – feelings, behaviour, sensorium
- Temporal features
- Attribution
- Causes, associated disorders
- Effects, coping
- Recapitulate.

SUGGESTED APPROACH

Patients often find depersonalisation and derealisation difficult to describe. They may admit to having them because they have misunderstood the question. Hence, it is important to ask for specific examples.

C : *Your doctor has asked me to look at some unpleasant experiences you have been having. Is that all right with you?*

Could you please explain what the problem is?

Depersonalisation

C : *Do you ever feel unreal?*

Have you ever felt as if you were outside of your body, watching a movie of yourself?

Have you felt as if you were far away from what was happening to you?

Do you sometimes feel as if you are living in a dream?

Have you ever felt as if your body or parts of your body were unreal or foreign?

Have you ever felt as if parts of your body were disconnected from the rest?

Do you sometimes feel like a robot or your movements mechanical or automatic?

When you cry or laugh, has it happened as if you do not feel any emotions at all?

Do you actually see, hear and experience them or feel them in your mind?

Can you describe it, please?

Derealisation

C : *Do you ever feel that things around you are unreal?*

Have you ever felt as if your surroundings were unreal, or artificial, like a stage set, with cardboard figures instead of real houses or trees?

Have you noticed any changes in the passage of time?

Can you give me an example?

Accompanying symptoms

C : *Does anything else happen when you have these experiences?*

How would you feel in yourself when these happen?

Are you able to think clearly when these happen?

Do your thoughts get muddled up when you have these experiences?

Temporal features

C : *When do these experiences occur?*

Do they happen when you are anxious or when you are relaxed?

How often does this happen?

How long would these usually last?

How long have you been having these problems?

Attribution

C : *What do you think might be causing these experiences?*

Is there some outside force or people causing them?

Are these things really happening or could they be just your imagination?

Causes, associated disorders

C : *Have you had any other mental health problems?*

Do you have thoughts coming into your mind against your will?

Do you have to check, count or do things repeatedly?

How do you feel in yourself most of the time?

Is there someone or something trying to harm you or make your life miserable?

Can you tell me about your drug habits?

Effects, coping

C : *How do these problems affect you?*

Do they make you feel frightened?

Do they affect your relationships or work?

How do you cope with these problems?

What have you done about them?

What do you think we should do?

Is there anything else you would like to tell me concerning these experiences?

Is there anything else we have to talk about?

Recapitulate

C : *Let me summarise what you have told me. Please tell me whether I have understood your experiences properly.*

44 Assess depression

L. Kissane

CONSTRUCT

The candidate demonstrates the ability to establish a rapport with a depressed patient and elicit the signs and symptoms and assess the severity of depression.

INSTRUCTIONS TO CANDIDATE

A GP has referred a middle-aged woman with a history of low mood. Do a diagnostic assessment and elicit symptoms of depression.

CHECKLIST

- Mood: depression, anxiety, irritability
- Biological symptoms: sleep, appetite, weight, energy, libido, diurnal variation
- Other symptoms: concentration, interests, anhedonia, self-esteem, obsessions
- Psychotic symptoms
- Suicide risk: hopelessness, guilt, death wishes, suicidal ideas, plans, preparation, acts
- Duration, causes
- Effect, coping and supports
- Insight
- Discuss diagnosis and treatment options
- Look for and respond to non-verbal cues.

SUGGESTED APPROACH

Mood

C : *Your doctor has asked me to see you because he is concerned about the way you feel in yourself. Could you please tell me how you feel?*

Can you describe it please?

Is it the same feeling that you have when something bad happens?

How is it different?

Have you cried at all?

Do you feel the same way every day?

What part of the day is the worst?

How difficult is it for you to snap out of this?

How anxious do you feel in yourself?

Ask about psychological and physical symptoms of anxiety and panic attacks.

Have you been feeling more irritable than usual recently?

Do you keep it to yourself?

How do you show it?

Biological symptoms

C : *How has your sleep been lately?*

Can you describe it?

How long does it take you to fall asleep?

Once you fall asleep, would you sleep until you wake up in the morning?

Has there been any change in the time you wake up in the morning?

How has your appetite been lately?

Has your weight changed recently? How much?

How have your energy levels been recently?

How does it affect you?

Have there been any changes in your sexual life recently?

Have there been any changes in your periods?

Other symptoms

C : *Can you think clearly?*

Do your thoughts tend to be muddled or slow?

What has your concentration been like recently?

Can you watch a TV programme right through?

How has your memory been?

Tell me about your interest in your usual activities and hobbies?

Do you enjoy things as much as you used to?

Can you enjoy being with your family or friends?

When did you last really enjoy something?

Have you wanted to stay away from other people?

How do you consider yourself compared to others?

How confident do you feel in yourself?

Do you find it difficult to make decisions even about everyday things?

Do you get awful thoughts coming into your mind even when you try to keep them out?

Do you spend a lot of time washing and cleaning?

Do you have to keep checking things again and again?

How have you been getting on with your day-to-day chores?

Psychotic symptoms

Nihilistic, hypochondriacal and persecutory delusions, auditory hallucinations.

C : *How's your health?*

Do you feel something terrible has happened or will happen to you?

Do you feel that you have to do something to save your family?

Do you hear people talking to you when you are alone?

Is there someone trying to harm you or make your life miserable?

Have you had any unusual experiences that you can't explain?

Do you have any regrets?

Do you feel you have done something wrong?

Do you blame yourself for anything?

Do you feel you deserve punishment?

Do you blame anyone else for your problems?

Suicide risk

C : *How do you see the future?*

Have you felt that life is not worth living?

Do you feel that you would be better off dead?

Would you do anything to harm yourself or hurt yourself?

What do you think you might do?

Have you made any plans?

How long have you been thinking about it?

Have you made any preparations?

Have you told anybody about it?

Have you done anything of that sort?

Duration, causes, effects, coping

C : *How long have you been feeling like this?*

What do you think might have caused this?

How is it affecting your life?

Has your work suffered because of this?

Has it affected your family?

How is it affecting your children?

How do you manage to cope?

Sometimes people tend to drink too much when they feel so bad. What about you?

Do you get any help?

What about family and friends?

What do you think has happened to you?

Have you had any treatment?

Is there anything else that we have to talk about?

What do you think is the problem?

What do you think we need to do about it?

Let me tell you what I think. You seem to have an illness called depression. Have you considered this possibility at all?

Let me explain. Depression is a common illness. However, it is a very treatable illness. We can treat your depression with medication and certain psychological treatments. Before that we need to do a physical examination and a few blood tests. I will give you some written material on depression and its treatments.

What do you think?

Explain hyperventilation and panic attacks

45

J. Anderson

CONSTRUCT

The candidate demonstrates the ability to establish a rapport with a patient and to explain how hyperventilation can cause panic attacks.

INSTRUCTIONS TO CANDIDATE:

A young woman has presented to A & E with panic attacks of 1 week duration. She has been on antidepressants for mixed anxiety and depression for the past month. The panic attacks started in the background of a worsening domestic situation. Explain how hyperventilation can cause panic attacks.

CHECKLIST

- Focus on the task
- Take a brief description of the panic attacks
- Explore the relationship between hyperventilation and panic attacks
- Explain management options
- Summarise.

SUGGESTED APPROACH

C : *I am Dr ____ , the psychiatric duty doctor. I understand that the casualty doctor has diagnosed that you had a panic attack. I have come to have a brief chat with you about it. Is that okay with you?*

P : Yes.

C : *First, could you describe an attack, please?*

P : I notice some chest discomfort. Then I know that it is coming. It takes me over. Once it is over, I am exhausted. Then I worry when the next one is coming.

C : *That is a good description. Can you explain a bit more about how it starts?*

P : The first thing I notice is some discomfort in my chest, or an unusual heart beat or I feel dizzy. This might come for no reason. Sometimes when I sit down for some time and then stand up, I feel dizzy. Then I know that it is coming.

C : *What happens in your mind when you know it is coming?*

P : I get a terrible fear, a terror. It is so dreadful. I worry that I might collapse or have a heart attack or die. My heart starts thumping. I feel dizzy. My chest feels constricted. I feel like choking. I get bathed in sweat. My body trembles. I get a tingling sensation in my arms and legs.

C : *What happens to your breathing?*

P : I feel breathless and dizzy. I feel choked. I rush out for some fresh air. I start breathing very fast – but why is it important?

157

C : *Normally when we are very frightened, our body responds so that we can either defend ourselves – 'fight' – or run away – 'flight'. The body has to increase the amount of oxygen supplied to the muscles and does so by breathing quickly. This is known as 'over-breathing' or hyperventilation. Do you notice fast shallow breaths and feel your chest moving?* [Put your hand at the top of your sternum so the patient is aware of where you are talking about.]

P : Yes, you are right, and then I fear that I will collapse or die.

C : *Often that fear makes the symptoms worse. With the increased oxygen that you breathe in, you are breathing out more carbon dioxide. Low levels of carbon dioxide will cause strange physical sensations such as dizziness, tinnitus, headache and a feeling of weakness. It can also cause faintness, numbness and tingling sensations in your hands and feet. Strangely enough, it also causes a feeling of breathlessness and that in turn makes you breathe faster, worsening and prolonging the attack.*

P : If that is correct, if I sit here and breathe very fast, I should get a panic attack.

C : *You are most likely to get one. In fact, I usually ask people with panic attacks to hyperventilate, so that they can understand how hyperventilating can start a panic attack. We cannot do that now because you should not drive for at least half an hour after having a panic attack. Moreover, if we do a blood test while you are having a panic attack, it is likely to show a low carbon dioxide level.*

P : Yes, I can see how that explains many of my symptoms, but why does this happen in the first place?

C : *It is quite likely that something in your surroundings triggered a thought, which you might not be aware of, but it was enough to set off the physiological response. You become aware of the physical symptoms. This makes you worry, for example, about whether you are going to have a heart attack, increasing your level of fear, and then the physiological response rapidly escalates. Can you see how it sets up a vicious circle?*

P : Are you saying that if I do not hyperventilate, I will not get a panic attack?

C : *Not exactly. What I am saying is that many patients with panic attacks hyperventilate. Hyperventilation can often start a panic attack and make an attack worse. By controlling your breathing, you may be able to reduce the unpleasant symptoms of hyperventilation, therefore bringing down the severity of attacks, shortening the attacks, and sometimes even aborting an attack.*

P : That is interesting. So what do I do about it?

C : *There are two things you can do. Some people breathe into a paper bag or cupped hands like this.* [Demonstrate by cupping your hands over your mouth and nose.] *Others avoid getting into the vicious circle by learning to control their breathing.*

P : So how can I learn this controlled breathing?

C : *There are a few different ways.*

We have an Anxiety Management Training Group, where we teach controlled breathing. There you will also learn muscle relaxation to counteract the sweating and shaking. If you don't like groups, we can teach you these in a one-to-one setting. The other option is for you to borrow our anxiety management and relaxation training video and audio tapes.

Another option is to make another longer appointment. I can show you how hyperventilation causes panic attacks and how you can control your breathing. Then you can try to learn the rest using one or more of the options we discussed just now.

I will give you an information leaflet explaining the various treatments on offer. This also explains how coffee, tea, coke etc. can make panic attacks worse, and other useful information. Does that make sense to you?

P : Yes. Thank you.

C : *We will have to talk briefly about other treatments also. Panic attacks can occur alone, called panic disorder. Or they may occur as part of anxiety, depression, phobias etc. In that case, we need to treat those disorders.*

For panic disorder as such, we usually use antidepressant drugs, cognitive behavioural therapy or both.

Is there anything else you would like to discuss with me?

P : No thanks.

C : *Let me summarise what we have discussed. You have a problem with panic attacks. It is likely that hyperventilating precipitates some of your panic attacks and also makes them worse. Therefore, we can control the panic attacks by controlling your breathing. You can learn to control your breathing by attending the anxiety management or relaxation training, in groups or one-to-one or using video or audio tapes. If you prefer we can make another appointment to show you how hyperventilation causes panic attacks and to learn controlled breathing. Please read this information leaflet and let us know what you would like to do.*

The main treatments used for panic attacks are antidepressant drugs or cognitive behavioural therapy or both. Even though panic attacks can occur on their own, they can be part of anxiety, depression or phobias.

46 Explain antidepressant medication

T. G. Dinan

CONSTRUCT

The candidate demonstrates the ability to establish a rapport with a patient with recurrent depression and to explain antidepressant treatment.

INSTRUCTIONS TO CANDIDATE

Explain antidepressant medication to a 22-year-old single mother with a 3-year history of recurrent depression. She relapses on drug discontinuation. She wants to have a baby with her current boyfriend. She wants to discuss with you about stopping the medication.

CHECKLIST

- Empathy
- Explain depression
- Explain need for medication
- Mechanism of action
- Pregnancy
- Breast-feeding
- Side effects
- How long to take medication.

SUGGESTED APPROACH

C : *I gather that you want to discuss your medication. Am I right?*

P : Yes, you are. First of all I want to clarify a few things. Isn't depression just the result of bad things happening to us?

C : *Of course, bad things that have happened in the past or happening now can make us depressed. But some people are more likely to get depressed than others, given similar circumstances. This can be due to genetic factors, or a traumatic childhood or a variety of other factors.*

P : Do I really need to take tablets? My mate told me that I should pull myself together.

C : *That is a good question. The issue is the difference between feeling sad and having the illness named depression. We all have times when we are feeling down or upset. They usually don't last a long time and may even prompt us to do things we need to do. Of course, we don't need medication for times like this, which are part of everyday life.*

On the other hand, the illness called depression is quite different. This makes one feel depressed, trapped, hopeless, guilty and even suicidal. It can affect one's concentration, motivation and ability to enjoy life. It also causes physical symptoms like poor sleep, loss of appetite, weight loss, lethargy and lack of sex drive. This does not go away. One cannot pull oneself together and get out of it. Unless treated it goes on for months, if not longer.

P : Will I get better with the medication?

C : *Seven out of every ten depressed people will get better on antidepressants. There are a number of other things which would help your recovery and reduce the chances of relapses, for example, having someone you can talk to, taking regular exercise, not drinking excess alcohol, eating well and using self-help techniques to help you relax.*

P : Why is it that I get better with medication, but then it comes back?

C : *It is very likely that your depression will come back if you stop the medication soon after getting better. For most people it will help them to prevent the depression coming back if they stay on the medication for up to a year or so after getting better.*

Some people experience severe depression again and again. Even when they have got better they may need to take antidepressants for several years, to stop their depression coming back.

P : How do they work?

C : *When depressed, some of the chemicals in the brain do not work properly. The antidepressants normalise these chemicals and thus make the depression lift. It can take 2 to 6 weeks or more to get completely better. It is very important to go on taking antidepressants every day during this time to get the full effect.*

P : My friend says that when she was young she got antidepressants for bed wetting. What else are antidepressants used for?

C : *Antidepressants are effective in treating a number of different illnesses such as anxiety, panic attacks, obsessions, chronic pain, eating disorders and post-traumatic stress disorder.*

P : We are planning to have another baby. Will I have to take them when pregnant?

C : *It will be better for you to become pregnant after you have become settled and remained well for some time.*

It is in the first 3 months of pregnancy that the mother's medication affects babies most. Therefore, if possible we avoid all medication during this time. However, one has to weigh up the pros and cons. If you become very depressed we may have to go for medication. So far no antidepressant has been shown to have any adverse effect on the growing fetus. However, it may be safer to go for one of the older anti-depressants.

P : What about breast-feeding?

C : *A baby will get only a tiny amount of antidepressant from its mother's milk. Babies older than a few weeks have very effective kidneys and liver. They are able to break down and get rid of medicines in the normal way. So the risk to the baby is very small. On balance, bearing in mind all the advantages of breast-feeding, it seems best to carry on with it while taking antidepressants.*

P : Will I get hooked on to them?

C : *The answer is no. Antidepressants are not like sleeping tablets. You don't develop tolerance to them, needing to take higher and higher doses. You don't get craving. When stopping any antidepressant it will be prudent to reduce the dose and stop rather than stopping abruptly.*

P : I remember my father having antidepressants when he was a bit senile. He had terrible problems with his waterworks. What side effects should I look for?

C : *The antidepressants we had until the late 1980s had some difficult side effects, especially in older people. For example, the tricyclic antidepressants can cause blurred vision, dry mouth, constipation, difficulty passing water, drowsiness, faintness due to low blood pressure etc.*

These days we prefer the newer antidepressants, especially in the middle-aged and the elderly. The commonest group is called the SSRIs. They also have side effects, but they are much easier to tolerate.

P : Can I drive when I take the medication?

C : *There are two issues here. Firstly, the depression itself can make driving unsafe. Secondly, the medication: again, the older tricyclic antidepressants are likely to make driving difficult due to the sedation and blurred vision. With most new antidepressant drugs this will not be a problem.*

P : I have heard that antidepressants cause sexual problems.

C : *Again there are two aspects. Firstly, depression itself can cause sexual problems like loss of interest in sex and difficulty in having an orgasm. Antidepressant drugs also can cause similar problems. However, it is often possible to alter this by reducing the dose or changing over to another drug.*

P : Is it all right if I discuss this with my family?

C : *It will be very useful to discuss this with your family, friends and your doctor. I will give you some information leaflets on antidepressants. If you wish to see me again, alone or with your family, please make another appointment. In the meantime I will write to your doctor.*

Is there anything else we need to talk about?

P : No thank you.

Explain the Mental Health Act

A. Battersby

CONSTRUCT

The candidate demonstrates an understanding of the fundamental principles of the Mental Health Act (1983).

INSTRUCTION TO CANDIDATE

William, a medical student on the first day of his attachment in psychiatry, is concerned that some of the patients on the ward are detained against their will. Explain the basic principles of the Mental Health Act (1983) and its common uses.

CHECKLIST

- General principles
- Admission for assessment
- Admission for treatment
- Assessment under the Act
- Appeal
- Leave
- Treatment of physical illness
- Other sections
- Mental Health Act Commission
- Provide an overview and do not become lost in minutiae.

SUGGESTED APPROACH

C : *I gather that you are concerned that some patients are detained on the ward against their will. Am I right?*

W : Yes. It seems really awful.

C : *I appreciate your concern. To start with, would you like to tell me what you already know about the Mental Health Act (MHA)?*

W : I am sorry, I have not heard about it before.

C : *That's all right. In general in our society, we respect people's autonomy to make their own decisions even when these can be harmful to themselves.*

Sometimes mental illness can affect a person's judgement and capacity to make decisions, or may cause them to act in ways that can harm themselves or, rarely, other people. The Mental Health Act (1983) is to ensure the safety, protection and treatment of people with mental illness.

W : What if you are not sure if someone is mentally ill or not?

C : *We would first consider assessing the person in the community or as an informal in-patient. We would consider whether the patient needs to be detained in the interests of the patient's own health or safety or with a view to the protection of other people.*

We use Section 2 of the Act when we are of the opinion that a patient is suffering from a mental disorder of a nature or degree that warrants admission to hospital for assessment. Under Section 2, a patient can be detained for up to 28 days.

W : What about treating patients with a confirmed mental illness?

C : *Here also we first try to provide treatment in the community or as an informal in-patient. We consider whether detention is necessary in the interests of the patient's health and safety and the protection of others. We proceed with Section 3 of the MHA only if the patient's mental illness warrants in-patient treatment. A Section 3 detention can last up to 6 months. At the end of this period, this section can be renewed if the conditions for detention under Section 3 are still met.*

W : Who decides if a patient needs to be detained under the Act and how?

C : *When concerns are raised about a person, we try to assess, support and treat them in the community or as an informal, that is, a voluntary in-patient. If that is either not possible or not safe, then two doctors and an Approved Social Worker (ASW) do an assessment under the Act. One of the doctors should be approved under Section 12(2) of the Act as having special experience in the diagnosis and treat-ment of mental disorder. The other doctor, if possible, has had previous acquain-tance with the patient and is often the patient's GP. The two doctors make recommendations and the ASW makes the application for admission to hospital under the Act.*

W : Having three people is not a safeguard, as the other two will surely agree with the psychiatrist.

C : *Not at all. In an assessment for detention under the Act, each professional involved has to make sure that they are satisfied that it is right to do that. If the profes-sionals involved disagree, they discuss the case and make arrangements to safeguard the interests of the patient.*

W : What if the patient believes that the detention is unfair?

C : *In such situations, the patient can appeal to the hospital managers and/or to the Mental Health Review Tribunal (MHRT). An MHRT is an independent panel composed of a legal representative, a consultant psychiatrist and a lay member. They can discharge the patient from a section, as can the Responsible Medical Officer (RMO), the hospital managers and the nearest relative.*

W : What if the patient leaves hospital?

C : *If patients detained under the Act abscond, they can be returned to the hospital. The important fact is that patients detained, for example, under Section 2 or 3 do not usually stay in the hospital for the whole 28 days or 6 months.*

When they become better, we start with increasing periods of leave under Section 17. Section 17 can be authorised only by the RMO.

W : Does the Act cover people with physical illness as well?

C : *No, in general, you cannot treat physical illnesses under the Act. However, there are exceptions, for example when a physical illness gives rise to psychiatric disorders as in delirium, or when the psychiatric disorder leads to physical complications as in eating disorders, or when the treatment of a psychiatric disorder necessitates regular blood monitoring as in clozapine treatment.*

W : Are there any other sections of the Mental Health Act?

C : *Yes, there are many different types.*

For example, the police can use Section 136 to bring a person suspected of being mentally ill to a place of safety.

Section 3 has provision for the patient to receive statutory aftercare when he leaves hospital under Section 117.

There are various sections relating to medication, mentally disordered offenders, guardianship etc.

W : You talked about treatment earlier.

C : *As in any other case we try to obtain informed consent to treatment. Even if the patient refuses consent, treatment can be given under the Act. After 3 months, if the patient still refuses treatment, a Second Opinion Appointed Doctor (SOAD) must be asked to review the case. If the SOAD agrees with the management then we continue treatment even without the patient's consent*

W : Are there any other safeguards to ensure good practice?

C : *Yes, the Mental Health Act Commission reviews how hospitals are using the Act. They visit hospitals on a regular basis to interview detained patients. They appoint medical practitioners to give second opinions under the Act.*

W : Is there any written information available?

C : *The Act is published on the Internet. It will be useful to look at the Code of Practice. We have a copy on the ward. You are also welcome to attend an Assessment under the Mental Health Act or a Manager's hearing or an MHRT hearing.*

48 Assess testamentary capacity

B. A. Lawlor

CONSTRUCT

The candidate demonstrates the ability to establish a rapport with an elderly patient with mild Alzheimer's disease and assess her testamentary capacity.

INSTRUCTIONS TO CANDIDATE

You are asked by a solicitor to assess testamentary capacity for a 72-year-old woman who has mild Alzheimer's disease.

CHECKLIST

- Rapport, empathy and ability to put the patient at ease
- Appropriate introduction, demonstrating awareness of possible cognitive deficits
- Mental State Examination: mood, delusions, and a brief cognitive assessment
- Criteria for testamentary capacity.

SUGGESTED APPROACH

C : *Thanks for coming to see me today. Are you aware what this visit is about?*

P : No doctor, my daughter told me this morning that I had an appointment today.

C : *I understand that you have decided to make a will, and I wanted to talk to you about it today. Is that all right with you?*

P : Yes doctor, that's fine. It is something I have been meaning to do for some time.

C : *As you know, when making your will you will be making some important decisions, and I have been asked to make sure that you understand what it involves. We will have a general chat about making wills, and then perhaps talk about your situation. If you have any questions or comments, feel free to ask them.*

Firstly, could you explain to me what a will is?

P : It is a document that I will write up. It will say how I want to divide my belongings, between my family members.

C : *Tell me more about it and how you would go about it.*

P : I will go to my solicitor and tell him who I want to have what when I die. I will then sign the document when he has it ready. He will keep it until I die and will see that my instructions are carried out when I die.

C : *What if your situation changes before you die?*

P : I would go back to him and change it.

C : *What assets or belongings do you have to leave in your will?*

P : Not a lot, doctor. I own my house and my car.

C : *How much is your house worth?*

P : I wouldn't have a clue, doctor. It would be worth more than I paid for it 40 years ago, which was £2000.

C : *Could you give me an estimate of what it would be worth?*

P : Well I know 2 years ago my neighbour got £100 000 for hers, so I presume it would be something similar.

C : *Is there anything else?*

P : I do not think so.

C : *Any savings?*

P : I had a savings account years ago, but I haven't put anything in it for a long time.

C : *What about your pension?*

Knight (1992) proposed the following criteria to help determine testamentary capacity. The individual:

● Is aware of what a will constitutes
● Knows the general extent of their assets
● Must be aware of the people who might reasonably expect to benefit from the assets
● Must be free of delusional beliefs that might affect the distribution of assets
● Must not be under the influence of any drugs that tend to distort his mental capacity as far as making a will is concerned.

Use open questions initially, but you may have to use reminders and prompts. For example, if they cannot remember the names of family members but seem to be aware of them you could help them out. If they cannot put a value on their house you could give them a few choices. If they cannot remember the details of their income you could make some suggestions.

If there is something that they did not tell you spontaneously, but with prompting they remembered it, you should check it with them again at the end.

Assess in brief other aspects of the mental state and do a cognitive assessment. Remember that symptoms can fluctuate. For example, depressive illness may affect motivation and cognitive functioning, and hence testamentary capacity. When the mood improves, the patient's capacity may improve also.

If the patient lacks capacity, then it is important to determine the causative factors, and whether any of these might be reversible.

At the end of the assessment, thank the patient and explain that you will send a report to the solicitor. If the patient has capacity, you could tell them that from your point of view there should not be a problem. If the patient does not have capacity, it is probably best to refer her to the solicitor, where plans for alternatives can be made.

REFERENCE

Knight B 1992 Legal Aspects of Medical Practice (5th edn). Churchill Livingstone, Edinburgh

49 Risk assessment in puerperal disorder

F. Hynes

CONSTRUCT

The candidate demonstrates the ability to establish a rapport with a patient who has recently had a baby and to do a risk assessment.

INSTRUCTIONS TO CANDIDATE

A & E staff ask you to see a young woman who is 3 weeks postpartum and has presented saying there is something wrong with her baby boy. A & E staff feel she is unsafe to go home alone with a baby. Complete a risk assessment.

CHECKLIST

- Gather a full psychiatric history
- Look for risk factors
- Assess relationship to the baby
- Mental State Examination:
    - Affective or psychotic symptoms involving the baby
    - Suicidal and infanticidal thoughts
    - Cognitive functions
- Physical examination
- Evidence of neglecting the baby.

SUGGESTED APPROACH

The patient may be distressed, frightened and paranoid. Acknowledge her distress.

C : *Hello, I am Dr ____ . The casualty staff asked me to speak to you to see if I could help. You seem very upset today. Can you tell me what is wrong?*

Allow her to speak freely for the first few moments, noting her concerns.

Present illness

Weepiness, irritability, anxiety, perplexity, bewilderment, disorientation.

Negative thinking, e.g. personal inadequacy, and failure to function as a good mother.

Anxiety about the well-being of the baby.

Abnormal ideas about the baby, e.g. the baby is malformed, abnormal or evil.

Persecutory ideas about family, friends.

Lability of mood, behaviour and psychotic symptoms.

Tiredness, insomnia or loss of sleep, hard work.

Look for risk factors

Pregnancy: psychiatric and physical problems

C : *How did you get on generally during the pregnancy?*

Birth: obstetric complications

C : *Tell me about how the delivery went.*

Time:

- Maternity blues – 3–10 days
- Depression – 3 weeks
- Psychosis – 2 weeks.

Perinatal: severe maternity blues, physical problems.

Past psychiatric history.

Family psychiatric history.

Mother: older age, single, primigravida

Premorbid personality: high interpersonal sensitivity

Social supports: marital conflict, other stresses – financial, family etc.

C : *Who do you live with?*
Are you currently in a relationship?
Have there been any difficulties since the baby was born?
How are things between you and your partner/husband?

Relationship to the baby

C : *Please tell me about your baby.*
Could you tell me what your baby is like?
How do you feel about him?
How are you coping with the baby?
Does he have any problems?
Does he sleep well?
How do you feel when he wakes you up in the night?
Does he cry too much?
How do you feel when he cries?
Have you been losing your temper with the baby?
Do you at times wish that someone else looked after him?

Mental State examination

Look especially for:

- Evidence of self-neglect
- Psychomotor retardation, agitation, restlessness
- Weepiness, irritability, anxiety, perplexity, bewilderment
- Lability of mood, behaviour and psychotic symptoms
- Affective or psychotic symptoms involving the baby.

C : *Are you worried about the baby?*
Do you think there is something wrong with the baby?
Do you feel that the baby is ill/abnormal/evil/dead?

Are you worried that something strange is going on with the baby?

Are you worried that someone will take the baby away?

How do you feel about your friends and family?

Do you blame yourself for something you have done or thought?

Have you heard voices asking you to harm the baby?

Risk of harm to self and to the baby

C : *How do you feel in yourself?*

Have you felt that things have become hopeless?

Do you feel useless or worthless as a mother?

Do you feel trapped as a mother?

Have things got so bad that you wished you were not here?

Have you thought of doing something to yourself?

What would you do?

Have things got so bad that you wished you never had a baby?

Have you thought about giving up the baby for adoption?

Do you ever wish that something would happen to him?

Do you have worrying thoughts about the baby?

Do you feel that you need to do something to the baby?

Can you explain that, please?

Consider, for example, plans to kill the baby to save it from the world.

Cognitive function: disorientation, impaired concentration and distractibility.

Physical examination: self-neglect, dehydration.

Evidence of neglecting the baby.

Insight

C : *What do you think is the problem?*

Do you think you might be unwell?

Lots of mothers struggle and it seems that it is difficult for you to cope with everything right now. I think you would benefit from some help. What do you think?

Assess capacity to refuse treatment

50

J. Bellhouse

CONSTRUCT

The candidate demonstrates the ability to establish a rapport with a patient who wants to withdraw consent for major elective surgery, assess his capacity and advise the surgical team.

INSTRUCTIONS TO CANDIDATE

Mr Jones is a 57-year-old businessman admitted to a general surgical ward in your hospital. He had an ultrasound scan for upper GI discomfort. The scan picked up an abdominal aortic aneurysm of 8 cm diameter. He was admitted for an elective repair of the aneurysm. After the routine work-up and a reasonable night's sleep he has declined to go ahead with the operation. He wishes to leave the hospital. The surgeons have asked you for advice as to whether he can go, given he has already signed the consent form.

CHECKLIST

- Ascertain the facts of the case
- Introduce yourself to the patient and explain the purpose of your assessment
- Assess his capacity to consent/withhold consent for the operation
- If he lacks capacity, ascertain the mental disorder responsible for this
- Inform the surgical team of your opinion and their options.

SUGGESTED APPROACH

Speak to the surgeons to ascertain the facts of the case

C : *Hello, Mr T, I am Dr X, the psychiatric SHO. I am about to see Mr Jones. Can you tell me about his case please?*

Why was he admitted?

What is the current problem?

What operation do you think you need to do? What are the risks?

What is his prognosis if the operation is performed?

What is the natural history of his condition if the operation is not done?

Introduce yourself to the patient and explain the purpose of the interview

C : *Hello, Mr Jones, I am Dr X, one of the psychiatric doctors in this hospital. Mr T, the consultant surgeon looking after you at the moment, has asked me to see you as he is concerned by your decision not to go ahead with the operation. I understand that you have a swelling of the main blood vessel in your abdomen. Mr T believes that, on balance, the best course of action is to repair the swelling now rather than wait* *for an emergency to arise. Tell me how you understand the problem and the proposed operation.*

The patient's understanding of the overall problem
C : *Tell me what you understand about the nature of the problem in your abdomen.*
What do you understand will happen to this swelling in the future?

The patient's understanding of the nature of the proposed procedure
C : *Do you know what the surgeons think needs to happen?*
Have you ever had an operation before?
What have you been told about the anaesthetic that would be used?

The patient's understanding of the purpose of the procedure
C : *Why do you think that you need an operation?*
Why do the surgeons think that you need an operation?

The patient's understanding of the risks of the procedure
C : *Have you been told about the risks of having the operation?*
Do you think that it will be painful?
Is it possible that you may die?
Do you think that it may leave you with scars?

The patient's understanding of the risks of not having the procedure
C : *What do you think will happen if nothing is done?*
Do you think that you will get better if nothing is done?

Having ascertained the patient's level of understanding, give the relevant information where the patient does not understand it and ask again. Give the information in simple, clear terms and on a bit-by-bit basis, then assess whether he has understood it.

Does the patient believe the above information?
C : *Do you believe there is a problem with the main blood vessel in your abdomen?*
Do you believe that if the swelling is not operated on, it may burst and cause major problems?
Do you believe that you could die if the swelling was to burst?

Is the patient able to weigh the information in order to come to a decision?
C : *So after all that, can you tell me the pros and cons of the operation?*
Tell me why you have decided not to have the operation.

Ascertain the final decision
C : *We have had a detailed discussion of why the surgical team feels you need the operation. Tell me, what do you think now about having the operation?*
Do you think it would be better to go ahead?
Why not?

If the patient has the capacity to make the decision, tell the patient what you have decided and how things will proceed

C : *It seems to me that as you have a sufficient grasp of the facts, you are capable of making the decision as to whether you go ahead with the operation or not. The fact that we believe you are capable of making this decision does not necessarily mean that we believe that you have made the best possible decision.*

I think it is very important that you meet Mr T to discuss this again in the near future. I will speak to him about you getting another opportunity to meet him and discuss the problem you have in the near future.

I will let your GP know that the operation did not go ahead as planned as you decided in the end not to give consent.

You must discuss with the staff here on the ward the procedure for finalising your discharge. It may well be that the surgical team will ask you to sign a 'discharge against medical advice' form, which reflects the fact that, although you are free to make the decision, it is contrary to the advice of Mr T's team.

If you change your mind at any time, you should make an appointment to see Mr T.

Thank the patient.

If the patient has been attentive throughout the interview, has understood and believed the relevant information, is fully aware that emergency repair is rarely as successful as elective repair and that it carries a much higher mortality rate, including death before getting to A & E, and if he has made a decision not to go ahead at this time owing to the fact that he currently is well and is willing to take a chance with his health rather than electively undergo a painful and complex procedure, he has the capacity to withhold consent for the procedure. Given he has capacity, at this juncture there is little to be gained from a detailed psychiatric history.

Notes

An adult with capacity has the right to refuse an operation even at the risk of dying (*Re T (Adult: refusal of treatment)* [1992] 4 All England Law Reports 649). Clearly, in an elective situation where there is time to reflect and for the patient to change his mind, it is rarely necessary to override a decision. However, even elective operations can be performed without consent where the patient lacks capacity, where this is in the best interests of the patient (*Re F (Mental patient: sterilisation)* [1990] 2 AC 1). A competent adult can only be overridden in one situation, where the Mental Health Act (1983) allows treatment of a mental disorder without reference to the capacity of the individual.

The fact that written consent has been given does not mean that a capable adult cannot change his or her mind.

51 Collateral history in dementia

M. Moran

CONSTRUCT
The candidate demonstrates the ability to establish a rapport with the relative of a patient with suspected dementia and to obtain a collateral history in an organised and structured way.

INSTRUCTIONS TO CANDIDATE
Obtain a collateral history from a woman whose husband is suspected of having dementia.

CHECKLIST
- Sensitivity, empathy and rapport
- Cognitive, functional, behavioural, psychological and physical symptoms
- Onset and progression of the symptoms
- Risk assessment
- History: past medical, past psychiatric history, personal, family etc.

SUGGESTED APPROACH
C : *Good morning, my name is Dr ___ . As you know, your husband has been referred for assessment of his memory complaint. An important part of that assessment is to obtain detailed information from a close relative about his symptoms and how they affect him. Therefore, I have a few questions to ask you. Please feel free to interrupt me or ask me any questions.*

R : Thank you. I hope I can answer all your questions.

C : *The questions will be mainly about the kind of problems that your husband has been having, and how they affect him, so I am sure you will do fine. Some questions may not appear relevant to your husband, but they are part of our routine assessments of memory complaints.*

Please describe for me the problems your husband has been having.

R : He is just very forgetful, and can get quite flustered.

C : *Can you give me examples of his forgetfulness?*

R : He forgets things I have just told him. He asks me the same questions over and over again. He forgets where he leaves things and spends a lot of time searching for them.

C : *Anything else that you have noticed?*

R : I am a bit worried about his driving. He seems to lose his way or not recognise where he is. We were on holiday a few months ago and he could not find his way around at all. I had to go everywhere with him. That's when I decided he should have it checked out.

C : *Anything else you are concerned about?*

R : He seems very quiet, spends a lot of time alone or staring at the TV, but I don't think he's taking it in.

Cognitive functions

Enquire about symptoms in all cognitive domains.

Memory, short and long term. Does prompting or recognition help? Is it consistent or patchy?

Temporal disorientation, spatial disorientation.

Language difficulties, word-finding problems, dysphasia.

Comprehension.

Dyspraxia, dysgraphia, reading difficulties.

Visuospatial difficulties, agnosias.

Judgement, decision making.

Executive functioning, initiation planning etc.

C : *The memory problems that you describe – do they affect his ability to look after himself, or to do the things he used to?*

R : Oh yes, doctor. He seems unable to play golf, he has paid bills twice and I think he has forgotten his medication on a few occasions.

Establish the degree of functional decline

Enquire about behavioural and psychological symptoms.

There was a suggestion of him being withdrawn. Hence, enquire about symptoms of depression, apathy, anxiety, psychotic symptoms, visual hallucinations, frontal symptoms, sleep disturbance, repetitive behaviours etc.

Enquire briefly about any associated physical symptoms, sensory impairment, gait disturbance, Parkinsonism, weakness of limbs, incontinence, change in appetite etc.

Onset and progression

Enquire about the onset of these symptoms, whether it was sudden or gradual.

If sudden, was it related to any other event, e.g. physical or otherwise?

Differentiate between sudden onset and sudden recognition.

What symptoms were noticed first?

How have the symptoms progressed, e.g. slowly progressive versus stepwise?

Are there any fluctuations?

Are symptoms worse at night?

Do a risk assessment

Safety in the home, cooker etc.

Management of finances.

Inappropriate use of medication, e.g. forgetting to take them or taking too many.

Driving assessment (in brief).

Has he made a will?

Other relevant factors in the patient's history

Current medication.

Past medical history.

Past psychiatric history.

Family history – in detail: while a patient may deny a family history of Alzheimer's disease, a positive family history may become apparent if asked about 'senility' or confusion in later life.

Personal history and risk factors for dementia:

- Education
- Occupation
- Alcohol
- Head Injury
- Boxing
- Living situation.

Thank the relative for their help and explain what the plan is from there on.

C : *I would now like to see your husband again. We would like to perform some memory tests, blood tests and a brain scan. After that, we will invite you and your husband in to discuss the outcome of the assessment, and treatment options.*

Do you have any questions for me?

R : No thanks doctor.

Explain cognitive behaviour therapy

M. Robertson

CONSTRUCT
The candidate demonstrates the ability to establish a rapport with a patient and to explain what cognitive behaviour therapy (CBT) is and how it works.

INSTRUCTIONS TO CANDIDATE
A GP has referred a 30-year-old woman to you for CBT. She has a history of only partial response to two different antidepressant drugs. The patient wants to know more about CBT. Explain to the patient how CBT works.

CHECKLIST
- Avoid jargon and lecturing
- Explain the nature and management of depression
- Explain how CBT works
- Address the patient's concerns and misconceptions
- Avoid false reassurance
- Offer further information.

SUGGESTED APPROACH
C : *I understand your doctor has suggested that you try CBT for your depression?*

P : Yes. I have had two types of medication. They did not help me at all. My doctor suggested I see you for this 'CBT'. I don't know what it is.

C : *Well, could you please tell me how much you already know about CBT?*

P : My doctor told me that CBT is a talking treatment. If the tablets didn't help, how can a talking treatment help?

C : *I will explain. Please feel free to interrupt me.*

There are two main types of treatments for depression. One is the physical treatments such as medication or ECT and the other is the psychological or talking treatments. Cognitive behavioural therapy or CBT is one of the most commonly used psychological treatments.

P : So does it mean that an expert will basically tell me to 'pull yourself together'?

C : *Not at all. The therapist will work with you to identify the thinking and behavioural patterns that contribute to how you feel, and help you to make changes.*

When people are depressed, they often have negative thoughts about themselves, their future and the world in general. These thoughts come automatically into their minds. These negative thoughts or 'cognitions' undermine their self-confidence, make them feel even more depressed and lead to unhelpful behaviours.

Think about a person who habitually thinks 'If things don't go the way I expect them to, then all will be lost.' He will seldom be able to see anything in a positive light and will feel depressed about himself and his future. Because he is negative about things he will approach them in an unhelpful way and not really pursue anything positive. His world will become a continual frustration and disappointment. He will feel more and more depressed, which will affect the way he acts and thinks, and so the cycle goes on.

P : So what does CBT do?

C : *CBT helps people identify the thoughts or cognitions and behaviour patterns that lead to depressed feelings, which in turn feed into that vicious cycle. CBT helps the person work out different ways of thinking and behaving that in turn will help them cope better. The person with depression can then start to challenge the thoughts with a more realistic view of the situation. They can experiment with different sorts of behaviours to see if this improves their mood. This often involves keeping a diary of mood, thoughts and behaviour to see how they are linked, scheduling activities through the day and rating them for pleasure, and learning to recognise thinking errors.*

P : Is that all?

C : *CBT also helps people to look at their 'rules for living'. These are strong beliefs about how we should live our lives. We pick up these from others as well as from our own experiences. They influence our lives a great deal without us being aware of them. For example, one may grow up with the belief that 'I am good only if I am always successful'. This is unrealistic and impossible. If one sticks to this idea, one will feel worthless and frustrated. We will be prone to become depressed. This is because the reality of life is that we all fail sometimes. Demanding the impossible of oneself is likely to make one feel frustrated and low. CBT can help us become aware of our 'rules'. It also helps us develop rules that are more helpful.*

P : Will I have to lie on a couch and talk about my toilet training and bowels? How I got on with my parents when I was a baby?

C : *Not quite. CBT looks at 'here and now' issues rather than things from the past. It helps people to learn new methods of coping and solving problems, which they can use for the rest of their lives. This is even though negative automatic thoughts and rules for living are often formed in childhood.*

P : How long will the therapy go on?

C : *CBT usually lasts for 8 to 12 weeks. Usually there will be one session a week, each lasting about 50 minutes.*

P : How can anyone sort out my problems in such a short period?

C : *Well, it will be you sorting out your own problems with the help of the CBT therapist. The treatment works by you changing your thinking and behaviour patterns. This will need to happen over the long term. You may need to come in from time to time for 'check-up' sessions.*

The therapist will expect you to do 'homework' between sessions. The therapist will ask you to keep a diary of your thoughts, feelings and behaviours in the situations that you find stressful. You and the therapist will then work on how you might challenge these thoughts and replace them with others. In the latter part of treatment, you and the therapist will concentrate on the 'rules for living'.

P : Can you have CBT when you are taking antidepressants?

C : *Absolutely. The scientific evidence is that they enhance each other's effects.*

P :   I am not only depressed, I am very anxious too. Will that be a problem?

C :   *No, not at all. The two often go hand in hand. CBT particularly suits people who want to be actively involved in dealing with their problems. We use CBT techniques to treat both depression and anxiety.*

P :   Can CBT prevent depression coming back?

C :   *Yes, it can. CBT helps change the unhelpful ways of thinking and the rules for living. Hence, it is effective in reducing the chances of relapse. In fact, the last few sessions focus on relapse prevention.*

P :   Will a psychologist be seeing me?

C :   *Someone with special training and experience in CBT such as a psychologist, a nurse therapist, a psychiatric social worker or a psychiatrist will be seeing you.*

P :   Is it the same as counselling?

C :   *They are both talking treatments, although CBT is much more structured. However, there are some similarities; for example, some forms of counselling would involve problem solving, changing the way we look at the world etc.*

P :   What am I likely to gain from CBT?

C :   *Broadly speaking, there are three main areas. The most important is improvement in symptoms. The second is to explore and solve factors that make you vulnerable to becoming depressed and anxious. The third is to make you skilled in CBT techniques, so that you can solve future problems yourself without the help of a therapist.*

P :   By the time I get home, I would have forgotten most of what we discussed.

C :   *I will give you some written information on CBT. I will be happy to see you again if you wish. You can bring your partner too if you like.*

53 | Physical examination in alcoholism

M. London

CONSTRUCT
The candidate demonstrates the ability to do a focused physical examination in a patient with alcohol dependence.

INSTRUCTIONS TO CANDIDATE
A 42-year-old man has been admitted for alcohol detoxification. He had his last drink the previous night. Do a focused physical examination.

CHECKLIST
- General examination and withdrawal symptoms
- Nervous system
- Liver
- Wernicke–Korsakoff symptoms
- Other complications.

SUGGESTED APPROACH
Greet the patient by name, introduce yourself and explain your role.

Explain why you are doing the physical exam.

Before each step, explain what you are going to do.

General examination and withdrawal symptoms
- Tremulousness
- Sweating
- Pulse
- Blood pressure
- Tremor of outstretched arms
- Dupuytren's contracture
- Anaemia
- Clubbing
- Pedal oedema
- Scars/bruises.

Sensation
The aim is to rule out peripheral neuropathy.

Check arms and legs.

Check both sides.

Pinprick
Use disposable neurological pins. Do not use venepuncture needles.

Demonstrate the sensation to the patient on the sternum. Explain to the patient:

C : *This is sharp and this is blunt. Please close your eyes and say 'blunt' or 'sharp' when I touch you with one of them.*

Start from periphery to centre until sensation is detected.

Vibration

Do not vibrate the tuning fork audibly.

Apply the tuning fork firmly to a bony prominence.

Apply vibrating and not vibrating.

Check on nail beds, wrist and elbow.

Joint position sense

Explain to the patient with eyes open.

C : *This is up and this is down. Please say 'up' or 'down' when you sense any movement.*

Grasp the fingers at the sides.

Use fine movements.

Start from peripheral to proximal joints until sensation is detected.

Fine touch

Use fine touch, not tickling or stroking.

Stance

Ask the patient to stand up.

Rhomberg's test

Ask the patient to stand up with eyes open and heels together.

Marked swaying suggests cerebellar disease.

Ask the patient to close his eyes.

Swaying suggests posterior column involvement.

Gait

Ask the patient to walk across the room on toes only and then on heels only.

Tandem walking

Demonstrate to the patient and then ask him to walk with the heel touching the toe of the previous step.

Liver

Inspection

Palmar erythema.

Ask the patient to look up at the ceiling and look for jaundice in the sclera.

Dilated blood vessels on the trunk.

181

Gynaecomastia.

Testicular atrophy.

Spider naevi.

Distension of abdomen.

Palpation

C : *Is your tummy hurting anywhere?*

Is it all right if I examine your tummy?

Keep your hand parallel to the skin surface.

Palpate superficially, looking at the patient's face for distress.

C : *Can you take a few deep breaths, please?*

Move your fingers up towards the right hypochondrium.

You may feel the edge of the liver. See if it is tender. Check its consistency and how many centimetres it extends from the costal margin.

Percussion

The upper border of liver normally lies in the fourth intercostal space.

The lower border is at the costal margin.

If the abdomen is distended, look for shifting dullness.

Lateral gaze palsy, nystagmus on lateral gaze

See 'Examine cranial nerves'

Explain your findings and the need for blood tests, and thank the patient.

Explain schizophrenia

54

A. Michael

CONSTRUCT

The candidate demonstrates the ability to establish a rapport with a distressed relative of a patient recently diagnosed to have schizophrenia and to explain its nature, aetiology, signs and symptoms, treatment and outcomes. The candidate explains the situation in a way the relative understands. The candidate balances accurate and realistic information with instillation of hope.

INSTRUCTIONS TO CANDIDATE

John is a 20-year-old man. He is currently an in-patient on your ward. He is recovering from his first episode of schizophrenia. His mother wants to discuss John's illness with you. John has given you permission to speak to his mother.

CHECKLIST

- Empathy
- Explain nature of the illness
- Alleviate guilt
- Explain medication and other treatments
- Explain prognosis
- Avoid false reassurance
- Offer further sessions and ongoing support
- Focus on the task. Do not try to elicit the history of schizophrenia.

SUGGESTED APPROACH

C : *Thank you very much for making this appointment. I appreciate that this is a very stressful time for you. Your son has given me permission to talk to you about his illness. I am afraid today we have only a few minutes. Next time we will make a longer appointment. Please ask me questions and please feel free to interrupt me.*

R : I was told that John has schizophrenia. What is schizophrenia?

C : *Schizophrenia is a serious mental illness. It affects thinking, emotions and behaviour. It affects one person in every 100. It usually starts between the ages of 15 and 35 years. The illness often lasts for a long time and can be very disabling.*

R : What causes schizophrenia?

C : *No one yet knows for sure what causes schizophrenia. There seem to be a number of different causes.*

Schizophrenia tends to run in families. About one in ten people with schizophrenia have a parent with the illness. Genes provide about half the explanation. Some affected people have changes in the structure of their brain. Some others may have had viral infections during pregnancy or problems during birth. Using street drugs like ecstasy, LSD, amphetamines and cannabis can bring on schizophrenia, or trigger it off in someone with a predisposition. Growing up in inner cities seems to increase the chances of developing the illness. In people with schizophrenia, certain chemical messengers in the brain, called neurotransmitters, such as dopamine do not work correctly.

Stressful events, although they cannot cause schizophrenia, may bring the illness on. Long-term stress, such as family tensions, may also make it worse.

R : Is schizophrenia split mind?

C : *No. Many people believe that someone with schizophrenia can appear perfectly normal at one time and suddenly change to a different person and even to a violent murderer the next minute. This is not true.*

R : Doesn't schizophrenia make people unpredictable and dangerous?

C : *People who suffer from schizophrenia are rarely dangerous. They are no more unpredictable than anyone else. Any violent behaviour is usually sparked off by street drugs or alcohol. This is the same as for people who do not suffer from schizophrenia.*

R : Can families cause schizophrenia?

C : *At one time, people believed that disturbed parents and families caused schizophrenia. Research has proven that families cannot and do not cause schizophrenia.*

However, stressful events, or difficult relationships in the family, can sometimes trigger an episode of schizophrenia in someone who is otherwise likely to develop it because of genetic and other factors.

Moreover, if one already has schizophrenia, family tensions can make it worse. In such cases, specific family therapy helps resolve the problem.

R : Can you tell me about the medication for schizophrenia, please?

C : *Medication, called antipsychotics, or neuroleptics, is the main part of treatment of schizophrenia. They help to alleviate the most disturbing symptoms of the illness.*

The older drugs, or 'typical' antipsychotics, can cause side effects such as stiffness, shakiness, a type of restlessness called akathisia, sleepiness, blurring of vision, constipation etc. All these side effects are reversible, except tardive dyskinesia. Tardive dyskinesia affects one out of every twenty people and causes permanent abnormal movements, especially of mouth and tongue.

There are several new drugs called 'atypical' antipsychotics. They are less likely to cause stiffness, shakiness, akathisia and tardive dyskinesia, but they often cause weight gain and sexual problems.

R : How does the medication work?

C : *As we discussed earlier, the symptoms of schizophrenia appear to be caused by changes in certain chemical messengers in the brain, called neurotransmitters, especially dopamine and possibly serotonin and others. The medication works by regulating these chemicals.*

R : John has improved a great deal. How long will he have to continue the medication?

C : *The medication controls the symptoms and promotes recovery, but they do not cure the illness. The symptoms often tend to come back. This is much less likely to happen if he continues taking medication even when he feels well. For most people, the symptoms usually come back in about 6 months after stopping medication. A small* *number of people are able to stop medication with no ill effects. Most people, however, need to take maintenance therapy indefinitely, to prevent relapse.*

It is hard for people to take the medication every day. They may find it easier to take it as an injection taken once every 2, 3 or 4 weeks.

R : Will we get any support after discharge?

C : *The goal of treatment is to help the person resume a life that is as normal as possible. Medication is only one part of the treatment. Medication helps mainly with removing the symptoms. For the best outcome, everyone involved, including the person, the family, the community psychiatric team and others need to work together from an early stage.*

R : What is the community psychiatric team?

C : *The community psychiatric team includes nurses, social workers, psychologists, occupational therapists, physiotherapists and others who have different skills in assessing and enhancing the abilities of the affected person. These include help in understanding and coping with the condition, rebuilding confidence, tackling risk factors that could lead to recurrence of the illness, providing support to continue with education and employment, education about the disorder, and support and counselling for the emotional effects etc.*

R : How effective is treatment? What happens in the long term? Will my son be able to go back to university?

C : *We can't cure schizophrenia. We can only control the symptoms. Only about 20% of people with schizophrenia recover after being unwell for a few months. About 70% have longer and repeated episodes with in-between periods when they are relatively better. About 10% have severe and longer episodes and troublesome symptoms that will continue to interfere with their lives.*

The illness is likely to affect one's studies, work and social life. However, many people with schizophrenia live independently, and more and more people are able to work and to have families.

People with schizophrenia are more likely to live in poverty and isolation, be physically ill and to commit suicide. Good treatment can go a long way to prevent this.

R : Where can I find more information?

C : *I will get you an information leaflet on schizophrenia. It has a list of self-help and support groups, books and web sites with information for patients as well as carers.*

55 Assess risk of violence

J. Gojer

CONSTRUCT
The candidate demonstrates the ability to assess the risk of violence in a young man suffering from psychosis.

INSTRUCTIONS TO CANDIDATE
A young man with a diagnosis of paranoid schizophrenia is attending your outpatient clinic for a routine follow-up. He has a history of violence to others when unwell. Assess his current risk of harm to others.

CHECKLIST
- Empathy
- Psychotic symptoms
- Anger
- Substance misuse
- Plans, opportunities, targets
- Management.

SUGGESTED APPROACH

Hallucinations
Enquire about hallucinations, especially command hallucinations and hallucinations of a derogatory or threatening content.

Insight into hallucinatory experiences.

Possible triggers for them.

How does he cope with them?

Are they compelling him to act in particular ways or take matters into his own hands?

Ask directly about thoughts of wanting to act on such experiences with aggression.

Delusions
Explore delusions of persecution and reference.

How does he intend to deal with the alleged persecutors?

Enquire about delusions of passivity and control.

Does he feel helpless, trapped or controlled?

What does he want to do about it?

Are there bizarre delusions/ideas?

Are there thoughts of revenge or retribution?

Enquire about any erotomanic interests that are not being reciprocated, urges to act on them or behaviours such as spying, stalking, writing letters, making phone calls and hiring detectives.

Ask about relationships and jealousy.

Enquire about checking, spying, thoughts of or behaviour suggestive of hurting the partner or her alleged lovers.

Anger and irritability

Enquire about anger and irritability.

To whom is the anger directed?

How often is it expressed?

Is it associated with acts of violence to people, property or both?

What are the triggers for anger?

Is there remorse following the outburst?

Is the anger associated with drug or alcohol use?

Substance misuse

Enquire about current alcohol and drug use.

How do drugs and alcohol usually affect his irritability and aggressive behaviour?

Plans, opportunities, targets

How does he intend to harm?

Does he have access to weapons or chemicals?

Who is at risk?

How imminent is it?

How serious can it be?

Management

How amenable is the risk to therapeutic modification?

Enquire about his compliance with medication.

Have there been any recent changes in his medication?

Would he consider that he is unwell now?

Would he consider any changes in his medication?

What are his thoughts about in-patient treatment if needed?

Discuss with him your duty to inform the concerned people.

How often does he see a mental health worker?

How does he get on with the mental health services?

Discuss an MRI brain scan report

A. Mitchell

CONSTRUCT

The candidate demonstrates the ability to interpret a written magnetic resonance image (MRI) head report from a radiologist regarding a case of likely early-onset dementia and to explain the results to a concerned relative.

INSTRUCTIONS TO CANDIDATE

Your consultant referred a 60-year-old man admitted with memory complaints, Mini Mental State Examination score of 20, low mood and Hamilton Depression Rating Scale score of 15 for an MRI brain scan. The consultant radiologist has sent the following report:

'An MRI head was carried out using longitudinal relaxation (T1) and transverse relaxation (T2) planes. Results were compared with a normal scan taken 1 year previously. On T1 image there is enlargement of the CSF space, with pronounced ventricular enlargement beyond that expected in healthy ageing. There is atrophy of the cerebral cortex, more pronounced in the medial temporal lobes (entorhinal cortex) on a coronal view. On T2 imaging there are several small hyperintensities probably representing white matter lesions in the periventricular area. There is no indication of a focal lesion.'

The patient's daughter, Mrs Jones, asks to discuss this. The patient has given permission to discuss pertinent details.

CHECKLIST

- Differential diagnosis of memory complaints in later life
- Interpretation of MRI scan report
- Diagnosis and investigation of early-onset dementia
- Communication with a relative
- Dealing with medical uncertainty.

SUGGESTED APPROACH

R : I am concerned about my father's deterioration in memory and mood. What could cause this presentation?

C : *There are a large number of conditions that can cause problems in memory and mood. If we take mood first, it is not unusual for people to become demoralised because of isolation, bereavement or stress in later life. Sometimes this progresses to a form of clinical depression that requires treatment.*

Regarding memory, a number of conditions can cause a deterioration in memory in later life. Actually, a small deterioration is expected in most people as they age. However, your father may be suffering from a brain disease that makes this worse, or it could be an effect of being low in mood or related to other factors such as prescribed medication.

R : Isn't it unusual to develop memory problems before the age of 65 years?

C : *Yes, you are right. Most people who have memory problems develop difficulties after the age of 65 years. That said, depression can affect people at any age. Also, some conditions that affect the brain and hence cause memory problems can begin in the fifties or sixties.*

R : I am afraid he may be developing a permanent memory problem. Is this a rational worry?

C : *To be honest, it is reasonable to be concerned that he might have a slowly progressive brain condition. As you know, when these are severe these conditions are called dementias. The commonest form of dementia is Alzheimer's disease. However, I wouldn't assume your father is suffering from this condition without further information. In addition, there are a number of alternative ways of helping people with memory complaints, however serious.*

R : Why did you ask for the head scan?

C : *The MRI head scan is a scientific development beyond the standard X-ray of the brain. It detects tiny magnetic currents in the brain emitted by tissue with a high water content. It will show several changes that occur in dementia, as well as other rare conditions. We performed the scan to exclude some causes that might be irrelevant and to narrow the list of conditions that your father might be suffering.*

R : And what did the scan show?

C : *The results of the scan are quite technical but I can interpret them for you if you wish. As I mentioned earlier, many people have age-related memory problems and this is often accompanied by a degree of shrinkage of the brain – this is called atrophy. The results of this scan do show atrophy but also suggest a degree of shrinkage greater than we would expect from his age alone. The area responsible for memory seems particularly affected. This tells us that there is almost certainly a medical reason behind your father's memory complaints but it does not tell us exactly what the cause is. There were also some small areas that might suggest some damage to the smallest blood vessels in the brain, but only in certain areas. Again, these can be a feature of normal ageing. We need to continue our investigations before we can tell you more about the diagnosis. What we can say is that there is absolutely no indication of a tumour on this report.*

R : What further investigations would help in this situation?

C : *We will recheck your father's physical health with a thorough clinical examination. I would suggest we (or a psychologist on the team) perform some more advanced memory tests. This is because there may be subtle differences between depression, normal ageing, Alzheimer's disease and other causes. I would also suggest that other forms of brain scan are considered. These are time consuming but could provide more information. Equally importantly, we will observe your father's day-to-day progress on the ward, which will help clarify if he has problems in any other areas. Perhaps it would be worthwhile talking with his GP to see if he has noted any pattern to the recent deterioration.*

R : Is there anything I can do to prevent other family members suffering the same problem?

C : *That's a very hard question to answer satisfactorily. There are a number of risk factors for depression and a number of risk factors for memory problems. Unfortunately, few of them are genuinely reversible. Some evidence links vascular disease with both conditions and hence avoiding smoking and leading a healthy lifestyle may reduce the onset of these conditions in later life. You may have heard about research into medication (such as anti-inflammatory drugs) and preventing dementia – suffice it to say this has not yet been proven and more work needs to be done. For now the best advice is to recognise potential problems early and ask for medical help as soon as possible.*

R : Thanks for the information so far. Can you summarise for me?

C : *Yes, your father has been admitted for investigation of low mood and memory problems. Investigations are currently ongoing and we do not have a clear answer at this stage. You have done the right thing by admitting him to hospital. We asked for a head scan in order to clarify the diagnosis and it looks like there are some brain changes which might go some way to explaining his memory difficulties. This takes us some way forward but we still need to be looking into things a bit more before we can give him and the family a clear answer. I would be delighted to meet with you again in a few weeks to do this.*

FURTHER READING

Bosscher L, Scheltens P 2002 MRI of the medial temporal lobe for the diagnosis of Alzheimer's disease. In Qizilbash N et al (eds) Evidence-Based Dementia Practice. Blackwell, Oxford, pp 154–162

Jagust W, Thisted R, Devous MD et al 2001. SPECT perfusion imaging in the diagnosis of Alzheimer's disease: a clinical–pathologic study. Neurology 56: 950–956

Explain the management of obsessive-compulsive disorder

57

J. E. Muller, D. J. Stein

CONSTRUCT

The candidate demonstrates the ability to establish a rapport with the patient and explain the management of obsessive-compulsive disorder (OCD).

INSTRUCTIONS TO CANDIDATE

A 28-year old man was referred by his GP with a diagnosis of OCD. He has been using citalopram 20 mg daily for the past 5 weeks, but still has prominent OCD symptoms. Explain the management of OCD to him.

CHECKLIST

- Empathy
- Model of OCD
- Pharmacotherapy: Drugs, side effects, contraindications, dose, duration, augmentation
- Psychotherapy: CBT, exposure and response prevention
- Involvement of friends/family
- Offer ongoing support
- Further information.

SUGGESTED APPROACH

C : *I understand your GP has been treating you for OCD. Tell me about it please.*

P : Yes, I'm taking citalopram, but I don't know if this is what I'm supposed to be taking. My OCD is still as bad as it was before I started treatment.

C : *What is your 'model' of OCD?*

What do you think causes it, and how do you think it should be best treated?

P : From what my doctor told me, I understand that OCD involves changes in particular brain circuits. I really think that my obsessions and compulsions are a kind of short circuit. And I'm hoping that the medication will help fix that.

C : *Yes, a number of my patients use phrases like 'short circuit' to describe their experience. And there's also growing scientific data to support a view of OCD as a 'false alarm' that is triggered in certain brain areas, which can be reset with the help of medication and what we call cognitive behaviour therapy.*

P : I read on the Internet that all of the available SSRIs are effective for OCD. Then how does my GP decide which of these SSRIs to give me?

C : *The SSRIs are more or less equally effective for OCD, although some agents may work better for some people, as each is slightly different. Similarly, SSRIs have a generally*

191

similar side-effect profile, although again for some people a particular agent may turn out to be the best tolerated.

P : I felt nauseous on the medication at first, but somehow that's better now. Was that a side effect? What else should I be looking out for?

C : *The SSRIs can cause early side effects like nausea and headaches, and as in your case these typically go away over time. In the long run, people may notice other problems, including impaired sexual function and weight changes. In general SSRIs are safe and well tolerated, but do report all possible side effects to your GP or me.*

It is important to check with your doctor before taking any other medication, because some drugs including some herbal remedies can interact with SSRIs.

P : I've been on citalopram for 5 weeks now. I know that many people who go on antidepressants start to improve in the first few weeks. I'm getting worried that I don't see any positive effects yet.

C : *It's true that in depression the mood can lift quite early on after medication is started. However, response to medication in OCD is often slower than in depression, taking place over weeks to months. Therefore, in order to see whether a medication is going to work in OCD, one really has to give it some time, around 10–12 weeks. How much citalopram do you take?*

P : One 20 mg tablet every morning.

C : *In OCD, we usually need to use higher dosages of medication than in depression. We start the medication at lower doses in order to limit side effects. We aim for the dosage that best controls your OCD, but at the same time causes minimal side effects. We need to increase your SSRI depending on response and side effects, so I suggest that you increase your medication to two tablets per day from now on.*

P : How long will I have to take medication for?

C : *Let's give the SSRI 3 months to see if it helps you. If it works it should be continued for a year or more. This would depend partly on whether cognitive behaviour therapy is helpful for you, because continuing to practise its techniques when you discontinue medication gives you a better chance of remaining well. And if you discontinue the medication, do it gradually.*

P : Once I get better, can I decrease the dose of my antidepressant?

C : *The rule of thumb is to stick with the dose that got you better, for that is also the dose that should keep your symptoms under control.*

P : I read on the Internet that neuroleptics are useful in OCD.

C : *Serotonin plays an important role in OCD, but another neurochemical called dopamine may also be a key. The neuroleptics block dopamine, so can be used as an 'add-on' in certain cases. People who have OCD and tics, for example, sometimes need this combination. If this add-on strategy works, response is usually seen at low doses and occurs early on. However, neuroleptics when used alone are not effective in OCD.*

P : What will happen if I do not respond to my present medication?

C : *Well, I'm still hopeful that may not be the case. But if necessary, the next step would be to switch you to another SSRI, as people who don't respond to one or more SSRIs can still respond to another, as each is somewhat different. When a number of SSRIs fail, then combinations of drugs can be helpful. But medication forms only a part of* *the treatment of OCD. It might turn out that the best augmenting agent for your OCD is psychotherapy.*

P : What's that about?

C : *The therapy of choice is called cognitive behaviour therapy, or CBT for short. The two basic principles are exposure and response prevention. This entails setting up a hierarchy of stimuli (objects, situations) that people fear and then gradually practising getting comfortable even when facing these fears (and not performing one's compulsions). The hierarchy is such that one can start with things that are relatively easy to deal with, before working up to more powerful fears. As OCD is associated with anxiety, it's sometimes easiest for people with OCD to simply avoid certain objects and situations. CBT focuses on reversing this pattern. This isn't always an easy treatment for people to follow, because it does involve practising to relax in anxiety-provoking situations. What's really interesting though is that brain imaging studies show that both medication and CBT are able to decrease the 'false alarm' that is seen in OCD, so this kind of technique can ultimately have very powerful effects.*

P : Yes, I'm interested in learning these techniques.

C : *How is the OCD affecting other aspects of your life, such as work and home?*

P : Work is fine, as I do most of my compulsions after hours. At home, however, things are more difficult – I've been asking my mum and dad not to touch certain things, and this has led to a fair bit of friction.

C : *OCD often affects relationships with one's friends and family. It might be hard for them to understand your rituals, and they sometimes blame themselves and feel guilty or helpless. At the same time, it's important that your family also understand the principles of exposure and response prevention, and they may even be able to help 'coach' you through some things. A possibility is to bring your parents in, to give them some information on OCD, and to discuss ways in which they can help out. I can also give you the details of support groups available for family members of patients with OCD.*

P : I'll talk to them about coming in. Is there anything else I can do?

C : *You might want to make contact with the Obsessive Compulsive Foundation, which is a patient advocacy and education organization, as well as your local OCD support group. I can also recommend some books, Internet resources and self-help manuals that you might find useful. Do you have any other questions?*

P : Not that I can think of.

Interpret ECG and electrolytes

D. MacDougall

CONSTRUCT

A 23-year-old woman is admitted with an eating disorder. She has been binge-eating and making herself sick. She has also possibly been using diuretics.

Urea and electrolytes report

Na^+	126 mmol/l
K+	2.8 mmol/l
Urea	12.8 mmol/l
Creatinine	142 μmol/l

INSTRUCTIONS TO CANDIDATE

Comment on the ECG and lab report. What other electrolyte disturbances may exist? How should this patient be managed?

CHECKLIST

- Electrolyte changes in eating disorder
- ECG changes in eating disorder
- Management of the above.

SUGGESTED APPROACH

Urea and electrolytes

The U & E report shows hyponatraemia, hypokalaemia, and a high urea and creatinine. These are consistent with vomiting and purgative/diuretic abuse.

ECG

The ECG is regularly irregular with an ectopic beat after two sinus beats. The rate is about 66/min. The axis is normal. The P waves are normal. The PR interval is 0.12 s (three small squares), which is normal. The QRS complexes, ST segments and T waves are also normal.

The ectopic beats themselves are ventricular in origin (broad complex, i.e. QRS complex more than three small squares wide) and unifocal (the same shape each time). Atrial and ventricular arrhythmias are common in hypokalaemia, which can be minor or life threatening.

Other electrolyte disturbances

The patient is likely to be hypochloraemic. If she has been using diuretics, magnesium levels may be low and it would be worth checking the level. If vomiting has

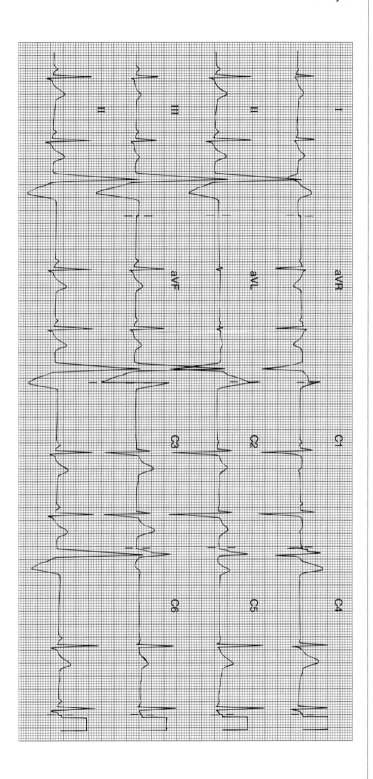

been significant or prolonged, the patient may have a metabolic alkalosis and hence I will measure bicarbonate and/or do a blood gas analysis.

Management

I will contact the medical registrar promptly and discuss how to correct the electrolyte abnormalities in this patient. Sodium and potassium need to be replaced. Intravenous normal saline with added potassium would be ideal, particularly if the patient won't comply with oral rehydration and potassium supplements. Replacement of potassium is particularly important in view of the ECG abnormality (multiple frequent ventricular ectopic beats). Ventricular ectopic beats themselves are not dangerous, but indicate an 'irritable' myocardium.

Elicit symptoms of grief

R. Jacob

CONSTRUCT

The candidate demonstrates the ability to establish a rapport with a recently bereaved person, elicit symptoms of grief and rule out symptoms of depression.

INSTRUCTIONS TO CANDIDATE

A GP has referred a 60-year-old man with a history of low mood of 3 months duration following the death of his son in a road traffic accident. Elicit symptoms of grief. Consider the possibility of a depressive disorder.

CHECKLIST

- Empathy
- The loss
- The reaction – look for features of normal versus pathological grief
- Rule out depressive symptoms
- Risk factors
- Supports
- Explanation.

SUGGESTED APPROACH

The loss

Enquire about the circumstances, duration, closeness of relationship, ambivalence, dependence etc.

C : *Your doctor has asked me to see you because he is concerned about you. I under-stand you have recently lost your son. I am very sorry. Are you able to talk about this?*

How long ago did this happen?

How did John die?

How old was John?

How did you and your son get on with each other?

I am sure that was the worst thing that has ever happened to you.

Is there someone to blame?

The reaction

Normal mourning: pangs of grief, angry pining, anxiety when confronted by reminders of loss, brief hallucinations, somatic symptoms, specific guilt, identification-related behaviours, acceptance, visiting grave.

Pathological: absent, delayed, prolonged mourning; excessive identification with, or idealisation of, the lost person, mummification, extreme denial, avoidance and self-reliance.

Health-related behaviours: excessive smoking and drinking.

Distorted grief refers to features other than depressive symptoms that are either unusual in degree, e.g. marked hostility, overactivity, extreme withdrawal, or in nature, e.g. physical symptoms that were part of the last illness of the deceased.

C : *How has John's death affected you?*

How do you feel about it now?

Do you think you have come to terms with your loss?

Do you feel angry?

Do you feel angry when something reminds you of John?

Do you blame yourself?

Do you feel guilty?

What do you feel guilty about?

How often do you visit John's grave?

Do you sometimes mistake strangers on the street for John?

Would you at times feel as if John is near you?

Sometimes when loved ones die, people keep their room and possessions as if they are still alive. What about you?

If the patient has feelings of presence, illusions or hallucinations, reassure and explain that they are not uncommon in normal grief reaction.

Depression

Look for retardation, generalised guilt, worthlessness, suicidal ideation after the first month, psychotic symptoms, severe functional impairment, hopelessness and wanting to join the deceased.

DSM-IV suggests diagnosing depression in the first 2 months only if severe functional impairment, worthlessness, suicidal ideation, retardation or psychotic symptoms are present.

Enquire about psychiatric history and medication.

Risk factors

Risk factors: sudden, unexpected, potentially stigmatised, due to negligence, multiple losses, pre-existing physical and mental health problems, low socio-economic status, lack of social supports.

C : *How has your health been lately?*

Have you had any other setbacks lately?

How do you spend your time?

Have you been back at work?

How has it affected your work?

Have you been smoking or drinking more than usual lately?

Supports

C : *Tell me about your family and friends, please.*

How do your wife and the rest of the family cope these days?

Are you able to discuss John's death with your family and friends?

Have you come across anyone else who has had a similar experience?

Do you find talking to them helpful?

What help have you been getting?

Do you keep in touch with your workmates and friends?

Do you think you have a problem and you need help?

Have you heard about CRUSE?

Explanation: *three options*

1. *I think you are going through a normal reaction to your tragedy. Any father in your position would be experiencing the same feelings. You are not mentally ill. As time passes you will start feeling better. However, with some help you will be able to cope even better.*

2. *It looks as though you have not been able to come to terms with your loss. Your loss seems to have an unusually severe effect on you. I think you will benefit from some counselling or talking to someone who knows exactly what you are going through.*

3. *I am afraid your grief has progressed into a depressive illness. This is a common problem. You will need grief counselling as well as treatment for depression. This could be psychological treatment, medication or both. These treatments will help you come out of your depression and grieve appropriately.*

C : *CRUSE Bereavement Care is a charity helping bereaved people to come to terms with their loss. I will give you their contact number. People generally find them very helpful.*

I would like to see you again in a month's time to make sure that everything is going all right. Is that okay with you?

If you need to see me before that, I will be happy to.

Is there anything else you would like to talk about?

I will write to your doctor about this.

If you wish, I will be happy to talk to your family about what we discussed.

60 Explain postnatal depression

A. Michael

CONSTRUCT

The candidate demonstrates the ability to establish a rapport with a pregnant woman who has a history of postnatal depression and explain the nature and prognosis of postnatal depression.

INSTRUCTIONS TO CANDIDATE

A 30-year-old woman who had postnatal depression following her first delivery has become pregnant again. She wants to talk to you about postnatal depression and the possibility of a relapse.

CHECKLIST

- Empathy
- Use non-medical language
- Allow her to express her concerns
- Risks
- Preventive measures
- Avoid false reassurance
- Further information and future contact.

SUGGESTED APPROACH

C : *How can I help you?*

P : I had depression after my first delivery. I am pregnant now. I want to talk about it.

C : *That's very sensible of you. It is always good to know and be prepared. I am afraid we have only 10 minutes today. You are welcome to make another longer appointment. Please feel free to interrupt me. Where would you like to start?*

P : Can you tell me what postnatal depression is?

C : *Postnatal depression, or PND for short, means becoming depressed after having a baby. One out of every ten women suffers PND. It usually starts within a month of the delivery but can start up to 6 months later. It can go on for months, or even years, if untreated.*

P : Is it not the same as baby blues?

C : *PND is a lot different from baby blues. Every other woman would feel a bit weepy, flat and unsure of herself on the third or fourth day after having a baby. We call this 'baby blues' or 'maternity blues'. This soon passes. Many women are weary and a bit disorganised when they get home from hospital, but they usually feel on top of the situation in a week or so. However, if it gets worse or lasts more than 2 weeks we have to consider PND.*

P : I can't remember what symptoms I had.

C : *PND is like any other depression. The mother feels weepy, anxious, low, unhappy, wretched and hopeless. She may feel irritable towards other children, occasionally to the baby and especially to the partner. She feels utterly exhausted and fatigued. She may have difficulty falling asleep and may wake up early. She may lose her appetite. She cannot enjoy things that used to be of interest and pleasure, including sex. She may feel unable to cope with the baby, unable to handle and feed the baby and may feel guilty about it. She may worry about the baby's health.*

P : What causes PND?

C : *No one knows of any one particular cause. One thing is sure. It is not because one is not cut out to be a mother or because one is ungrateful or unmotherly.*

There are certain things which may increase the risk of getting PND, such as a previous history of depression, lack of support from the partner, a premature or otherwise ailing baby, the mother's loss of her own mother when she was a child and an accumulation of misfortunes, for example bereavement, the partner losing his job, housing and money problems. However, a woman can suffer from PND when none of these applies and there is no obvious reason at all.

P : Could it be hormonal?

C : *Huge hormone changes take place at the time of giving birth. Levels of oestrogen, progesterone and other hormones to do with reproduction, which may also affect emotions, drop suddenly after the baby is born. However, women who do and who do not get PND have similar hormone changes.*

P : Would mothers with PND harm the baby?

C : *No, they don't. In fact, many mothers, even those without any mental health problems, can sometimes feel like 'throwing the screaming monster out of the window'. Mothers with PND often worry that they might harm their babies, but they never do.*

However, there is another postnatal illness called puerperal psychosis, when there is a risk of the mother harming the baby. In this illness, the mother may be convinced the baby is evil or that the only way of saving the baby from some imagined misery is to end its life. Fortunately, this is a much rarer condition, affecting only two out of every 1000 mothers.

P : What treatments are available?

C : *Since PND is similar to depression occurring at other times, the treatment is also similar. Often, the mother may need only reassurance, practical support and supportive counselling. We have self-help and support groups available locally. They encourage mutual support and advice regarding mothering, childcare and dealing with depression. If depression is associated with marital or housing problems, they will have to be tackled. For some, antidepressant drugs will be needed. In very severe cases, other drugs and even ECT may be needed. Another aspect of treatment is educating new fathers about PND and helping them to adjust.*

P : Can I breast-feed when taking the medication?

C : *Yes. You need not necessarily stop breast-feeding. We can find an antidepressant that does not get into your milk and affect your baby in any way.*

P : How long will I have to continue the medication?

C : *In the case of women with the first episode of PND, it will be best to continue the medication for at least 6 months after the depression has lifted.*

P : Can I have hormone treatment instead of antidepressants?

C : *Hormones appeal to many women more than antidepressants, because they seem more 'natural'. However, the evidence that they work is less impressive, and they are not necessarily harmless, for example, if there is a history of blood clots.*

P : What would happen if a mother gets PND and she does not take any treatment?

C : *Most women will get better after 2 to 6 months. In some, it may last even a year or two. However, this means a lot of suffering. PND can affect mothering, bonding and the relationship with the baby's father. Hence, it is best to diagnose and treat it as early as possible.*

P : What are the chances of me getting PND this time?

C : *The chance of someone without a history of depression getting PND is 10–15% and for someone who had one episode of PND getting a second one is 20–40%.*

P : Is there any way to prevent it?

C : *We don't know enough about PND in order to prevent it. However, common sense would suggest to moderate commitments, to look after oneself with respect to nutrition, exercise, rest, sleep and company, attend antenatal classes and keep in touch with the GP, antenatal clinic and health visitor etc. Some researchers have found that psycho-education and support programmes can halve the chances of getting a second PND. Most importantly, if there is any doubt that you may be getting PND, seek help immediately.*

P : Can PND in the mother affect the baby?

C : *There is research evidence that PND adversely affects the mother–infant relationship and the cognitive and emotional development of the infant. That is why we have to diagnose and treat PND as early as possible. However, evidence on the consequences in early childhood is less clear.*

P : I can't think of any more questions.

C : *I will give you some literature on PND. It also has information about some useful books and web sites. Please contact me if there is any problem. I will try to see you as soon as possible.*

Index

Printed in Great Britain
by Amazon.co.uk, Ltd.,
Marston Gate.